Student's Atlas of
NEUROANATOMY

Walter J. Hendelman, M.D., C.M.
Professor
Department of Anatomy and Microbiology
Faculty of Medicine
University of Ottawa
Ottawa, Ontario, Canada

Student's Atlas of
NEUROANATOMY

W.B. SAUNDERS COMPANY
A Division of Harcourt Brace & Company
Philadelphia London Toronto Montreal Sydney Tokyo

W.B. SAUNDERS COMPANY
A Division of Harcourt Brace & Company

The Curtis Center
Independence Square West
Philadelphia, Pennsylvania 19106

Library of Congress Cataloging-in-Publication Data

Hendelman, Walter.
    Student's atlas of neuroanatomy/Walter J. Hendelman.
       p.   cm.
    ISBN 0–7216–5428–2
    1. Neuroanatomy—Atlases. I. Title.
    [DNLM: 1. Brain—anatomy & histology—atlases. 2. Spinal Cord—
anatomy & histology—atlases. WL 17 H495s 1994]
    QM451.H35 1994
    611′.81—dc20
    DNLM/DLC   93-41702

Student's Atlas of Neuroanatomy   ISBN 0–7216–5428–2

The 1988 and 1987 editions were originally published by University of Ottawa Press.

Printed in the United States of America

Last digit is the print number: 9   8   7   6   5   4   3   2

Preface

The educational goal of this Atlas is to assist the student in understanding the functional anatomy of the human central nervous system.

The idea of creating an atlas of neuroanatomy for students was based on my experience as a teacher of medical students. I often found the task very difficult, if not frustrating. Most texts and atlases seem to be directed at a more specialized student (or have been written, so it seems, for colleagues). Was there not a better or simpler way to gain an understanding of the complex three-dimensional structures of the human brain? Could there not be an atlas with illustrations containing core or essential information tailored for the beginning student?

After a chance meeting with some interested second-year medical students who were taking the course offered in our medical faculty, one talented person (Mr. Jean-Pierre Morrissey) was subsequently hired as a summer student to create some drawings of some of the more difficult portions (e.g., the brain stem). While conceiving the diagrams and deciding what to include, the content of the *Atlas* was also being determined. It became immediately apparent that explanatory text should accompany each illustration. And thus the *Atlas* was born! The University of Ottawa Press undertook to publish it and did so in an exceedingly short timeframe (in September, 1987).

The original drawings were created so that the student could color various structures or pathways, as instructed (e.g., Section B and Parts C-I and C-II). This was done from an educational perspective in order to make the book "interactive," as well as to keep the publication costs low. In fact, those students who add the color actually seem to learn by doing, and the final product has more depth and information. It has therefore been decided to retain this feature of the *Atlas*. The subsequent inclusion of photographic material, some of it special dissections that have been found useful in teaching, led to the publication of the second edition of the *Atlas* a year later.

The present (third) edition has been a few years in the making. It was my good fortune to meet up with a very talented medically trained graduate student, Dr. Andrei Rosen, who accepted the challenge of creating some illustrations on the limbic system, one of the most difficult subsets of structures of the brain to capture. These drawings were done using an air brush technique and have a unique three-dimensional perspective. We then went on to create other diagrams: on the basal ganglia, the thalamus, and the pathways of the brain stem. In all, about thirty new diagrams have been added to this third edition, some replacing others from the previous editions.

The basic orientation of the *Atlas* has been maintained—to present the material from the perspective of a student learning the subject matter for the first time. Each drawing has explanatory text containing "core" information; this has been extensively revised and now includes functional and clinically relevant commentary. In addition, there is frequent cross-referencing, so that the student is guided to other diagrams that show the same structure. Although the *Atlas* is meant to accompany a course with a text and/or lecture notes, it can be used by a student for self-study in a problem-based curriculum.

The organization of the *Atlas* is as follows: the cerebral hemispheres are presented at the beginning, first the cortical aspects and then structures found within. The brain stem (and cranial nerves) is considered next, followed by sensory and motor pathways. Then the thalamus is presented, with the cerebellum next, and finally the spinal cord. The limbic system is placed at the end of the *Atlas* since not all courses on the central nervous system would discuss this set of brain structures. A glossary of terms has also been added.

Although the target audience of this *Atlas* is the medical student, students in the allied health sciences (nursing, occupational therapy, and physiotherapy) who require a knowledge of the nervous system should find this *Atlas* quite useful; this may also include graduate (or undergraduate) students in a neuroscience program. Residents in neurology, neurosurgery, physiatry, and psychiatry may also find some of the illustrations quite instructive, particularly those on the brain stem and its pathways and those on the limbic system.

Creating this *Atlas* has been a most enjoyable experience for me. I hope that you, the student, will derive similar pleasure from learning about the human brain. I believe that the subject matter is inherently fascinating and worth the effort required to understand it.

WALTER J. HENDELMAN, M.D., C.M.

Acknowledgments

This *Atlas* could not have been created without the efforts and contributions of the following:

Illustrations

Mr. Jean-Pierre Morrissey, medical student, now graduated (Sections B, E, and F and Parts C-I and C-II)

Dr. Andrei Rosen (M.D.), currently a graduate student in the Faculty of Medicine, University of Ottawa (Part A-II, Part C-III, Sections D and G)

Photography

Mr. Stanley Klosevych, formerly Director of the Health Sciences Communication Services, University of Ottawa, now retired (photographic material mainly in Part A-I)

Mr. Robert Lacombe, Health Sciences Communication Services, University of Ottawa (color photographs of the brain stem cross sections)

Medical Artist

Mr. Emil Purgina, Health Sciences Communication Services, University of Ottawa (artistic advice and labeling; Fig. 11)

The effort of the staff of the University of Ottawa Press, who undertook the publication of the earlier editions, is gratefully acknowledged. These editions were supported in part by grants from the Teaching Resources Service of the University of Ottawa.

The author appreciates the feedback that he received from medical and occupational therapy students who have used the *Atlas* over the years. This has helped in shaping the present edition and correcting some errors.

The support of the Department of Anatomy and Neurobiology of the University of Ottawa is gratefully acknowledged. Mr. Michael Simmons of the prosector staff prepared some of the dissections shown in the photographs.

I would like to express a special thanks to the staff of W. B. Saunders, particularly Mr. Lawrence McGrew, who caringly brought this edition to publication.

WALTER J. HENDELMAN, M.D., C.M.

Instructions for Color Coding

NOTE TO THE STUDENT: You are encouraged to color in the diagrams as instructed, particularly those on the brain stem cross sections (Section B) and the diagrams of the various pathways (Section C, Parts I and II), for the following reasons:

1. The color adds information and depth to these diagrams.
2. While doing the coloring, you are actively engaged in identifying the structure, and this contributes to the learning process.
3. Using the colors as instructed adds functional significance, for example, light blue for sensory cranial nerve nuclei.

Structure	Number	Color
Section A-II		
Basal ganglia		Light green
Thalamus		Red
Ventricles		Dark blue
Sections B, C, and D		
Background		Yellow
Miscellaneous		Orange
Red nucleus	3	Red
Ascending sensory tracts	4	Pink
Vestibular, MLF	5	Purple
Descending motor tracts	6	Dark blue
Cranial nerve nuclei—sensory (also locus ceruleus)	7	Light blue
Vision	8	Light green
Cerebellum-related	9	Dark green
Cranial nerve nuclei—motor	10	Light brown
Auditory	11	Dark brown
Substantia nigra	12	Black
Section F		
Nuclei and tracts—sensory		Pink
Nuclei and tracts—motor		Dark blue
Miscellaneous		Orange

Depending on your learning style, you may wish to use a colored marker or highlighter with some of the other diagrams in the *Atlas*.

Contents

SECTION C
Pathways of the Central Nervous System   91

SECTION D
The Thalamus   127

SECTION E
The Cerebellum   143

SECTION F
The Spinal Cord
159

Introduction, 159

SECTION G
The Limbic System
175

Introduction, 175

Introduction

The central nervous system (CNS) is composed of neurons and supporting cells, the glia. Neuronal membranes are specialized for electrochemical events, which allows these cells to receive, transmit, and communicate messages to other neurons. Anatomically, the dendrites and cell bodies of the neurons receive information, and the axons transmit the firing pattern of the cell to the next neuron. Communication occurs for the most part at specialized junctions called *synapses*.

Within the CNS, neurons that share a common function are often grouped together; such collections are called *nuclei*. Another way of separating neurons functionally is by arranging the cells in layers, whereby cells in different layers have different functions. Cells forming layers are usually located on the outer aspect of the brain's surface, and the whole arrangement is called a *cortex*. The cerebral cortex is the major functional cortex with six layers; the cerebellum also has a cortex, with three layers. Few areas within the brain are layered.

Much of the remainder of the brain consists of axons that connect one part of the brain with other areas. These fibers link the various parts of the brain with one another. Many of the axons are myelinated.

There are two types of glial cells: *astrocytes* are involved in supportive metabolic events, and *oligodendrocytes* aid in the maintenance of myelin, which ensheaths some of the axons.

Living brain tissue does not have a firm consistency, and the brain needs to be fixed for gross and microscopic examination. One of the most common fixatives used to preserve tissue is formalin. Nervous tissue fixed in formalin can be handled and sectioned. Areas containing predominantly neuronal cell bodies (and their dendrites and synapses) become grayish after formalin fixation, and this is traditionally called *gray matter*. Tracts containing myelinated axons become white with formalin fixation, and such areas are likewise simply called the *white matter*.

Organization of the Central Nervous System

The nervous system has evolved from a simpler to a more complex organizational network of cells.

The basic unit of the CNS is the spinal cord. The incoming sensory nerves and the outgoing motor nerves organize the spinal cord into segments (e.g., cervical, lumbar). Reflex circuits and other motor patterns are organized in the spinal cord. Afferent and efferent information concerning the autonomic nervous system is also part of the functioning of the spinal cord. (The spinal cord is described in Section F.)

As the systems of the brain become more complex, new control "centers" have evolved. These are often spoken of as higher centers. The first of these is located in the brain stem, which includes the medulla, pons, and midbrain (described in Section B and seen in photographic view in Fig. 21 and diagrammatically on the front cover and in Fig. 70). Groups of cells within the brain stem are concerned with essential functions such as the regulation of blood pressure, pulse, and respiration. Other groups of cells within the brain

1

stem are involved in setting our level of arousal, and play an important role in maintaining our state of consciousness. Special nuclei in the brain stem are responsible for some basic types of movements in response to gravity or sound. In addition, most of the cranial nerves and their nuclei are anchored in the brain stem. Many nuclei in the brain stem are related to the cerebellum.

The cerebellum is situated behind the brain stem (as in Figs. 12, 21, and 22 and on the front cover). This part of the brain is involved in motor coordination and in the planning of movements. Parts of the cerebellum are quite old in the evolutionary sense, and parts are relatively newer. This is reflected by the diverse connections of the cerebellum with the rest of the CNS. (The cerebellum is discussed in Section E.) The cerebellum has a simpler form of cortex that consists of only three layers.

Next in the hierarchy of the development of the CNS is the area of the brain called the *diencephalon* (see Figs. 22, 52, and 70). Its largest part, the *thalamus,* develops in conjunction with the next part, the *cerebral hemispheres.* (The thalamus is described in Section D.) Its smallest part, the *hypothalamus,* serves mostly as part of the neuroendocrine system, giving rise to neurohormones that regulate the cells of the anterior and posterior pituitary. It is also the *head ganglion* of the autonomic nervous system. Parts of the hypothalamus are intimately connected with the expression of basic drives (e.g., hunger and thirst) and with "emotional" behavior (see later discussion).

With the continued evolution of the brain, encephalization has occurred, culminating in the development of the *cerebral hemispheres.* Buried within the cerebral hemispheres are the basal ganglia, large collections of neurons (see Fig. 12) involved mainly in the initiation and organization of motor movements. These neurons affect motor activity through their influence on the cerebral cortex. (The basal ganglia are described in Part A-II.)

One of the major morphologic and organizational shifts was the formation of the six-layered cerebral cortex, the *neocortex.* The neurons occupy the outside surface and are organized in layers. In humans, the cerebral cortex is thrown into ridges and valleys (gyri and sulci), which allows for a greater amount of cortical tissue to occupy the inside of the skull (the cranial cavity). The expansion of the cerebral cortex in humans, both in terms of size and complexity, has resulted in this part of the brain becoming the dominant controller of the CNS, being capable, so it seems, of overriding most of the other regulatory systems. (The various cortical areas are described in the first section of the *Atlas.*) The cerebral cortex is necessary for thinking, consciousness, language, and many other functions related to the sensory and motor systems.

A number of areas of the brain are involved in behavior characterized by the reaction of the animal or person to situations. This reaction is often termed "emotional" and in humans consists of both psychological and physiologic changes. Various parts of the brain are involved with these activities; collectively, they have been named the *limbic system.* This network of neurons includes those found in specific regions of the cortex, various subcortical areas, parts of the basal ganglia, the hypothalamus, and parts of the brain stem. (The limbic system is described in the final section of the *Atlas;* see Section G and Figs. 70 and 71.)

For the nervous system to function properly, communication must occur between the various parts. Some of these communicative links are the major sensory and motor pathways, called *tracts* (or *fasciculi*—described in Section C). Much of the mass of brain tissue is made up of these axonal bundles. One of the major puzzles in the growth and development of the nervous system involves how the various parts of the nervous system link up with one another in a seemingly precise manner. Some of the early maturation in infants and children can be accounted for by the progressive myelination of the various pathways within the CNS.

Cerebral Hemispheres: Cerebral Cortex, Basal Ganglia, and Ventricles

INTRODUCTION

Cerebral Cortex (Part A-I)

The brains of the higher apes and humans are dominated by the cerebral hemispheres. Their size and complexity have made them the object of intense study. The nervous tissue of the hemispheres is responsible for consciousness, language, thinking, memory, movement, sensory perception, and certain aspects of emotion. In short, neuronal processing in the hemispheres to a large extent determines our capabilities. This is not to say that the other parts of the central nervous system (CNS) are not important, but working in and adapting to our complex modern world depends on the proper functioning of the cerebral hemispheres.

The hemispheres are organized in the following way. The neurons and their dendrites are grouped together on the surface to form a *cortex*. In formalin-fixed material, this takes on a grayish appearance and is often referred to as the gray matter. Most of the cerebral cortex is *neocortex*, because the neurons are organized in six layers, with each layer having a different function. Different areas of the cerebral cortex are functionally distinct, and this is reflected in the histologic differences between the areas. Some parts have a predominantly motor function, whereas other parts are receiving areas for one of the major sensory systems. Most of the cerebral cortex in humans has an "association function," which can be explained as serving to interrelate the various activities in the different parts of the brain.

One of the other major features of the cerebral cortex is the number of neurons devoted to communicating with other neurons of the cortex. These interneurons are essential for the processing and elaboration of information, whether generated in the external world or internally by our "thoughts." This intercommunicating network is reflected in the vast interconnections between cortical areas. Therefore, the various bundles of axons that run within the hemispheres are discussed in this section, along with the cerebral cortex.

The axons are located within the depths of the hemispheres. They have a white coloration after fixation in formalin, and these regions are usually called the *white matter*. The white matter bundles within the hemispheres are of three kinds—those interconnecting the various cortical areas on the same side (*association bundles*), those connecting cortical areas across the midline (*commissural bundles*), and those connecting the cerebral cortex with various subcortical structures (*projection fibers*).

Internal Structures (Part A-II)

The structures that are found within the depths of the cerebral hemispheres include the basal ganglia, the cerebral ventricles, and the white matter bundles, particularly those connecting the cortex with subcortical structures in the diencephalon, brain stem, and spinal cord.

BASAL GANGLIA

As mentioned, within the hemispheres are large collections of neurons, the *basal ganglia*. These masses of neurons function in tandem with the cerebral cortex. They are best known for their role in movement disorders, such as Parkinson's disease and Huntington's chorea. Some parts of this neuronal mass are also known to be involved in cognitive (i.e., thinking) activities. In addition, other parts of the basal ganglia are functionally part of our "emotional brain," the limbic system.

In humans, the basal ganglia consist of three major nuclei and some associated nuclei. The principal nuclei have a complex arrangement in space, and visualization of their location requires an understanding of the cerebral ventricles.

VENTRICLES

Some parts of the original neural tube, from whose walls the CNS developed, are still present in the hemispheres; these are the *cerebral ventricles*. Their position and shape are important in understanding the anatomy of the internal structures of the cerebral hemispheres.

INTERNAL CAPSULE

The white matter bundles that course between parts of the basal ganglia and the diencephalon are collectively grouped together and called the *internal capsule*. These so-called projection fibers are axons going to and coming from the cerebral cortex, linking the cortex with the diencephalon, brain stem, and spinal cord.

Cerebral Blood Supply (Part A-III)

Study of the CNS is not complete without a good knowledge of the blood supply. Nervous tissue depends for its viability on the continuous supply of both oxygen and glucose. Failure of the blood supply to a region, either because of occlusion or hemorrhage, will lead to death of the neurons and axons, resulting in functional deficits. An understanding of the subsequent clinical syndromes requires a detailed knowledge of the structure and function of the CNS.

PART A–I

CORTEX AND WHITE MATTER (Photographic Views)
(Figures 1–9)

FIGURE 1   ### The Hemispheres: Dorsal View

The surface of the hemispheres in humans and some other species is thrown into irregular folds. These ridges are called *gyri* (singular, *gyrus*), and the intervening crevices are called *sulci* (singular, *sulcus*). A very deep sulcus is called a *fissure*. This arrangement allows for a greater surface area to be accommodated within the same space—that is, inside the cranial cavity.

The surface of the cerebral hemispheres can be visualized from a number of directions—from above (dorsal view), from the side (dorsolateral view), and from below (inferior view). In addition, after dividing the two hemispheres along the interhemispheric fissure (in the midline), the hemispheres are seen to have a medial surface as well.

This photograph is a view of the cerebral hemispheres from above, a dorsal view. The arachnoid and pia (parts of the meninges) have not been removed from this specimen, which means that the blood vessels are also present. Removing these meninges allows for a clearer view of the gyri and sulci (see Fig. 2). Under the arachnoid membrane is a space, the subarachnoid space, which is collapsed in this fixed specimen; it is normally filled with cerebrospinal fluid (CSF). The interhemispheric fissure is normally occupied by a dural sheath (the falx cerebri) and a large cerebral vein, called a dural venous sinus (the superior sagittal sinus), which collects blood from the veins draining the surface of the hemispheres.

Different parts of the cortex have different functions. Therefore, it is important to delineate anatomically the various functional areas of the cortex. This forms the basis for the understanding of the possible clinical implications of lesions in the various parts of the brain, a task becoming more sophisticated with the help of modern imaging techniques, such as computed tomography (CT) and magnetic resonance imaging (MRI).

The basic division of each of the hemispheres is into four lobes—frontal, parietal, temporal, and occipital. Two prominent fissures—the *central fissure* and the *lateral fissure*—allow this subdivision to be made. The central fissure, which is easier to identify on the right side of this specimen, divides the area anteriorly, which is the *frontal lobe,* from the area posteriorly, the *parietal lobe*. The parietal lobe extends posteriorly to the *parieto-occipital fissure,* which will be better seen on other views (see Fig. 7). The brain area behind this fissure is the *occipital lobe*. The temporal lobe and the lateral fissure cannot be seen on this view of the brain.

Functionally, major areas of the frontal lobes have a predominantly motor function. The most anterior parts of the frontal lobe are the newest in evolution and are known functionally as the *prefrontal area*. This broad cortical area seems to be the chief "executive" part of the brain. The parietal areas are connected to sensory inputs and have a major role in integrating sensory information from the various sensory systems. The occipital lobe is concerned with the processing of visual information.

This photographic view shows some coral-like whitish material lying adjacent to the interhemispheric fissure. This material is collectively called the *arachnoid granulations*. These are in fact collections of tiny arachnoid villi. These villi are small outcroppings of the subarachnoid space that protrude through the dura and into the venous sinuses, thereby allowing the CSF to be reabsorbed from the subarachnoid space into the venous system (see Fig. 11).

Anterior

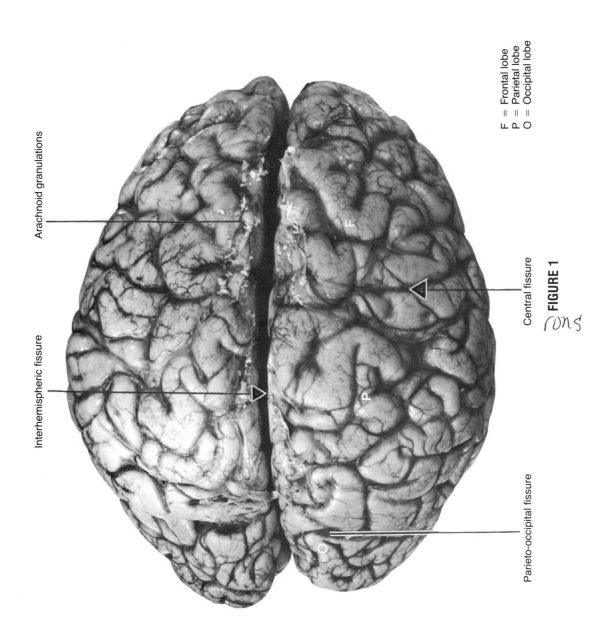

Arachnoid granulations

Interhemispheric fissure

F = Frontal lobe
P = Parietal lobe
O = Occipital lobe

Central fissure

Parieto-occipital fissure

FIGURE 1

runs

7

FIGURE 2

The Hemispheres: Dorsolateral View

With the meninges removed, it is possible to identify the sulci and fissures with more certainty. The central fissure (often called the *Rolandic fissure* or the *fissure of Rolando*) is now seen more completely, dividing the frontal lobe anteriorly from the parietal lobe posteriorly.

Some cortical areas are linked directly to either a sensory or a motor system; these are known as the *primary areas*. The gyrus in front of the central fissure is called the *precentral gyrus* (see Fig. 57) and is an area specialized for the control of movements. The gyrus behind the central fissure is the *postcentral gyrus* (see Fig. 54) and has a sensory function. An area in the frontal lobe (outlined) has a motor function in regard to eye movements; this is called the *frontal eye field*. (Other sensory primary areas will be identified at the appropriate time.)

Those cortical areas that are not directly linked to either a sensory or motor function are called the *association cortex*. The area in front of the frontal eye fields would be the prefrontal cortex, a typical example of an association area. Large parts of the parietal and temporal lobes are association cortex.

The cortex has been studied by many people using different techniques. It is possible to recognize distinctive morphologic (microscopic) features between different cortical areas, and these might reflect the differing functions of each particular area. One of the most commonly used subparcelations of the cerebral cortex is that of Brodmann, who divided brain areas numerically. Some of these numbers are sometimes used interchangeably with the names, such as area 4 for the precentral gyrus (the motor strip), area 8 for the frontal eye field, area 6 for a premotor strip between areas 4 and 8 (see Fig. 57), and areas 3, 1, and 2 for the postcentral sensory gyrus.

Some cortical functions are not equally divided between the two hemispheres. One hemisphere is therefore said to be *dominant* for that function. This is the case for language ability, which is located in the left hemisphere in most right-handed people. This photograph shows the right hemisphere, and the two language areas are indicated—*Broca's* area for the motor aspects and *Wernicke's area* for the comprehension of written and verbal language. The areas indicated on this brain specimen would presumably be responsible for language in a naturally left-handed person.

The lateral fissure (*fissure of Sylvius*) divides the *temporal lobe* below from the frontal and parietal lobes above. Extending the line of the lateral fissure posteriorly continues the demarcation between the temporal and parietal lobes. In the parietal lobe are two gyri—the *supramarginal* and *angular gyri*—whose association type of function is known. These areas, particularly on the nondominant side, seem to be involved in visuospatial activities. The specialized cortical areas for hearing are located within the lateral fissure (as shown in Fig. 3).

The location of the parieto-occipital fissure is indicated on this photograph (it is seen best on the medial view of the brain; see Fig. 7). This fissure separates the parietal lobe from the occipital lobe. The *cerebellum* lies below the occipital lobe, separated from it by dura, the *tentorium cerebelli*.

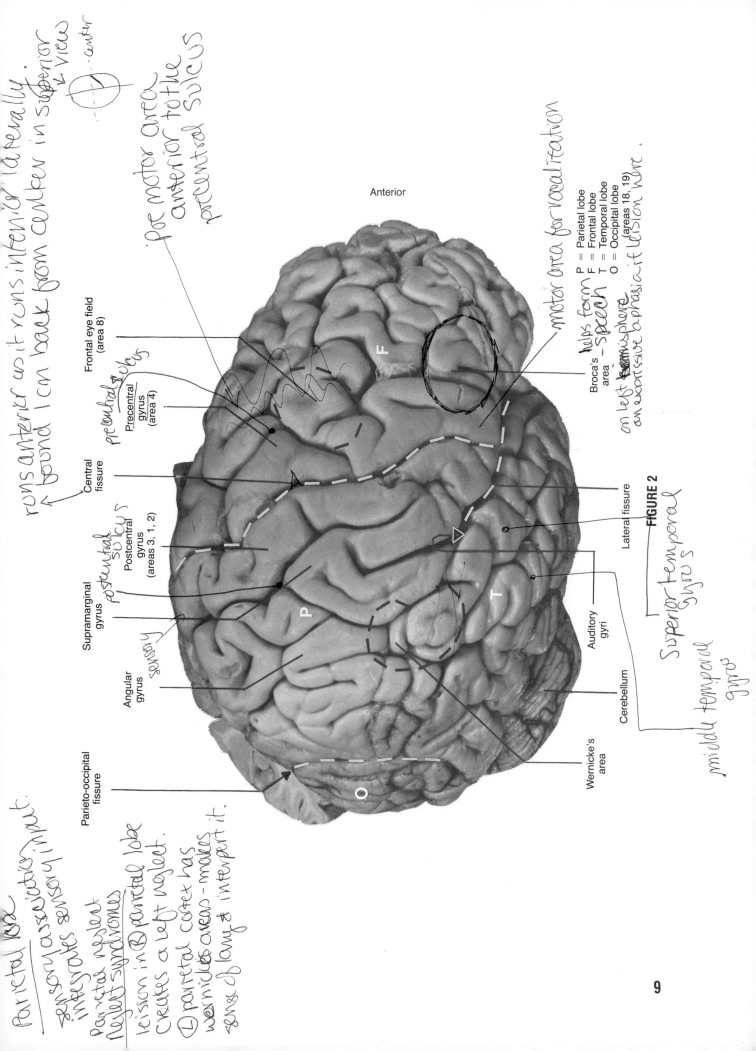

Anterior

Frontal eye field
(area 8)

Precentral
gyrus
(area 4)

Central
fissure

Supramarginal
gyrus

Postcentral
gyrus
(areas 3, 1, 2)

Angular
gyrus

Parieto-occipital
fissure

Lateral fissure

Auditory
gyri

Cerebellum

Wernicke's
area

P = Parietal lobe
F = Frontal lobe
T = Temporal lobe
O = Occipital lobe

Broca's
area

FIGURE 2

F

P

T

O

Handwritten annotations:

center

runs anterior wit runs interior laterally
← found 1 cm back from center in superior
view

per motor area
anterior to the
postcentral sulcus

Precentral sulcus

Postcentral sulcus

sensory

motor area for vocalization

helps form — speech

on left hemisphere
an expressive aphasia if lesion here.

Superior temporal
gyrus

middle temporal
gyrus

Parietal lobe
sensory/association input.
integrates sensory input.

Parietal neglect
neglect syndromes

lesion in ® parietal lobe
creates a left neglect.
⊕ parietal cortex has
wernickes areas — makes
sense of lang & interpret it.

FIGURE 3   # Auditory Gyri

The lateral fissure has been opened slightly, exposing two gyri oriented transversely. These gyri are the areas of the cortex that receive the incoming auditory sensory information first. They are named the *transverse gyri of Heschl* (see Fig. 55).

The lateral fissure forms a complete separation between this part of the temporal lobe and the frontal and parietal lobes above. Looked at descriptively, the auditory gyri occupy the superior aspect of the temporal lobe.

Further opening of the lateral fissure reveals some cortical tissue completely hidden from view. This area is called the *insula,* and a small part of it is seen in this photograph. It is important not to confuse the two areas, the auditory gyri and the insula.

Cortical representation of sensory systems reflects the particular sensation. The auditory gyri are organized according to pitch, giving rise to the term *tonotopic localization.* The postcentral gyrus has a representation of the body, with large cortical areas devoted to the hand and face. This is called *somatotopic localization;* this representation of the body has been given the name *sensory homunculus.* The precentral strip has an equivalent representation, the *motor homunculus,* again with large areas devoted to the hand and face, reflecting the fine control possible with these muscles.

The lateral fissure usually has within it a large number of blood vessels, branches of the middle cerebral artery. These branches emerge and then become distributed to the cortical tissue seen on the dorsolateral surface, including the frontal, temporal, parietal, and occipital cortices (discussed with Fig. 20).

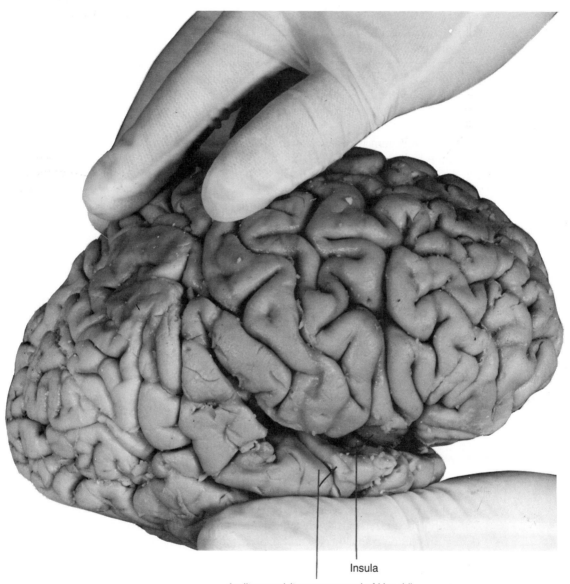

Insula

Auditory gyri (transverse gyri of Heschl)

FIGURE 3

FIGURE 4

The Hemispheres: Inferior Surface

This is a photographic view of the intact brain seen from below, which includes the brain stem and cerebellum. The medulla and pons, parts of the brain stem, can be identified, but the midbrain itself cannot be seen. The cranial nerves are still attached to the brain stem, and the arteries to the brain stem and cerebellum are also present.

The inferior surface of the frontal lobe extends from the frontal pole to the anterior tip of the temporal lobe (and the beginning of the lateral fissure.) These gyri rest on the roof of the orbit and are sometimes referred to as the *orbital gyri*. This cortex is again association type.

The next area is the inferior surface of the temporal lobe. The temporal lobes extend medially toward the midbrain and end in a blunt knob of tissue known as the *uncus*. Moving laterally from the uncus, the first sulcus visible is the *collateral sulcus*/fissure (seen clearly on the right side of this photograph). This demarcates the *parahippocampal gyrus*, which is the most medial gyrus of the temporal lobe; the uncus is the most medial protrusion of this gyrus. The parahippocampal gyrus is part of the limbic system (discussed with Figs. 70 and 75).

The cerebellum is more posterior, hidden in part by the brain stem. Above the cerebellum is the occipital lobe (as shown in Fig. 5; see also Fig. 7). In the space between the cerebellum and the hemispheres is a dural sheath, the tentorium cerebelli (not present on the specimen).

Several arteries are visible in this photograph. The two *vertebral* arteries unite to form the *basilar* artery (which is displaced from the midline of the pons in this specimen). The arterial supply to the brain stem and cerebellum comes from these arteries. There are three pairs of cerebellar arteries—*posterior inferior, anterior inferior,* and *superior*. The posterior inferior cerebellar artery branches off the vertebral artery. The anterior inferior cerebellar artery comes off the basilar artery (seen only on the right side on this specimen). The basilar artery gives off the two superior cerebellar arteries at the upper level of the pons, and ends by dividing into the *posterior cerebral arteries*. (The arterial circle of Willis is discussed with Figure 20.)

Various aspects of the cranial nerves are apparent here, starting with the *olfactory tract* on the inferior surface of the frontal lobe. The olfactory nerves penetrate the roof of the nose (the cribriform plate) and synapse in the *olfactory bulb* (discussed with Fig. 81). This is the bulbous enlargement seen at the anterior end of the olfactory tract. In the midline, just at the posterior edge of the frontal lobe, is the *optic chiasm*. Within the chiasm, there is a partial crossing (decussation) of the visual fibers (discussed with Fig. 56A). Posterior to this is the region of the hypothalamus, which will be seen more clearly in Figure 5.

Cranial nerve III, the *oculomotor nerve*, exits from the midbrain and is seen coursing between the posterior cerebral artery (rostral) and the superior cerebellar artery (caudal to it; seen clearly on the left side of the photograph). The *trigeminal nerve*, cranial nerve V, is located on the middle cerebellar peduncle (discussed with Figs. 23 and 24). Cranial nerves VII and VIII are seen attached to the brain stem at the pontocerebellar angle. (Further description of the cranial nerves and their attachments will be deferred to Section B.)

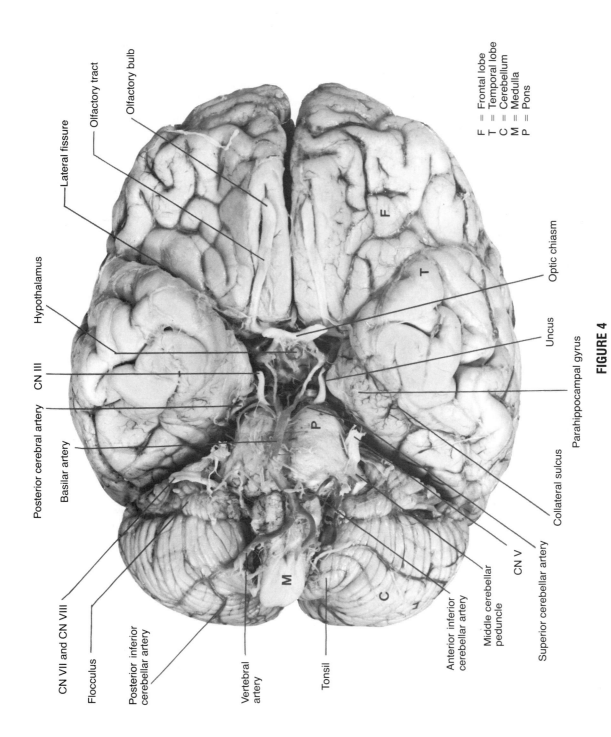

Olfactory tract

Olfactory bulb

Lateral fissure

F = Frontal lobe
T = Temporal lobe
C = Cerebellum
M = Medulla
P = Pons

F

T

Optic chiasm

Hypothalamus

CN III

Posterior cerebral artery

Basilar artery

Uncus

Parahippocampal gyrus

FIGURE 4

P

M

C

Collateral sulcus

CN VII and CN VIII

Flocculus

Posterior inferior cerebellar artery

Vertebral artery

Tonsil

Anterior inferior cerebellar artery

Middle cerebellar peduncle

CN V

Superior cerebellar artery

FIGURE 5

Inferior Surface: Brain Stem Removed

The brain stem has been sectioned through at the level of the midbrain, removing the brain stem itself and the attached cerebellum. The cut surface of the midbrain exposes for view the pigmented cells of the *substantia nigra* (discussed with the cross sections of the midbrain in Part B-II).

Removal of the brain stem and the cerebellum reveals the inferior surface of both the temporal and the occipital lobes. It is not possible to define the boundary between the two lobes on this view. The parahippocampal gyrus should be noted on both sides, with the collateral sulcus demarcating its lateral border. The uncus is clearly seen on both sides, with its blunted tips pointed medially.

The uncus lies just above the free edge of the tentorium cerebelli. The occurrence of a tumor, a large cerebral hemorrhage, or swelling of the brain for any reason leads to an increase in the mass of tissue in the cranial cavity and therefore to an increase in intracranial pressure. This causes the cerebral hemispheres to be displaced, pushing the brain downward. This pressure forces the brain through the tentorial notch, with the uncus at its leading edge. The whole process is referred to as *uncal herniation*. Because the edges of the tentorium cerebelli are rather rigid, the extra tissue in the area causes a compression of the brain matter, leading to brain stem compression and a progressive loss of consciousness. Cranial nerve III is usually compressed as well, damaging it and causing a fixed and dilated pupil on that side.

The *optic nerves* lead to the optic chiasm. Behind the optic chiasm is the *median eminence* and the *mammillary bodies,* both of which belong to the hypothalamus. The median eminence is an elevation of tissue that contains some hypothalamic nuclei. The pituitary stalk (not pictured here) is attached to the median eminence and connects the hypothalmus to the pituitary gland. The paired mammillary bodies are two nuclei of the hypothalamus (discussed with the limbic system, e.g., Fig. 73).

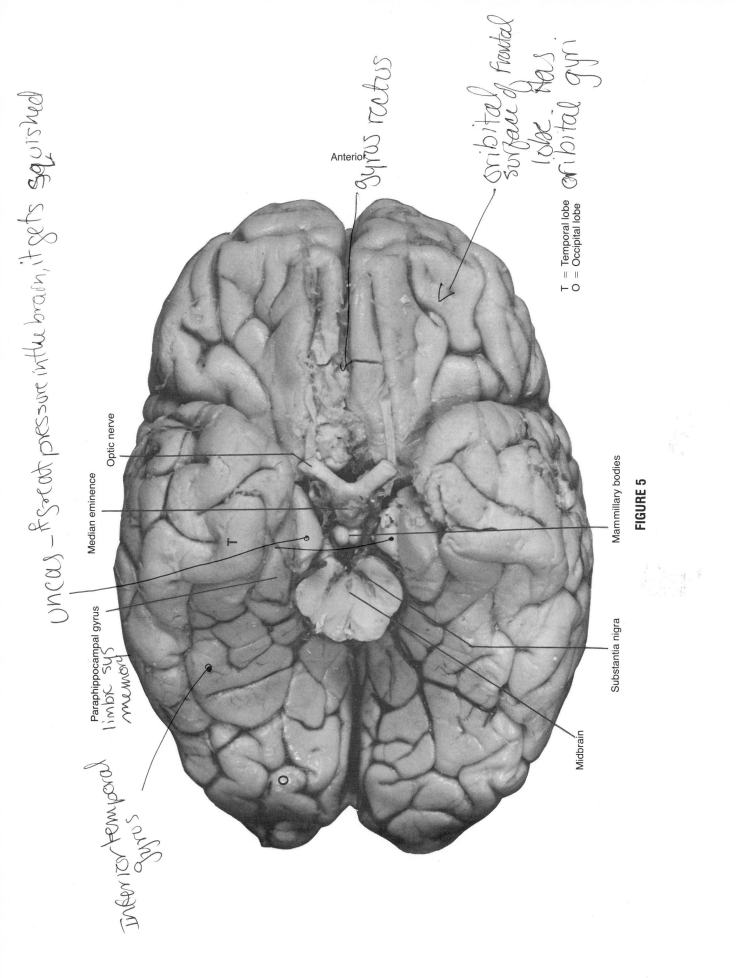

Uncus — if great pressure in the brain, it gets squished

gyrus rectus

Anterior

orbital frontal surface of frontal lobe - has orbital gyri

Optic nerve

Median eminence

Paraphippocampal gyrus
limbic sys
memory

Inferior temporal gyrus

T = Temporal lobe
O = Occipital lobe

Mammillary bodies

Substantia nigra

Midbrain

T

O

FIGURE 5

15

FIGURE 6 # The Corpus Callosum

The brain is again viewed from above. The superior sagittal venous sinus and the dura between the hemispheres, the falx cerebri, have been removed.

If the deep fissure between the two hemispheres is opened, the *corpus callosum* can be seen. This is a large bundle of axons (white matter) that cross the midline. Functionally, the axons connect one hemisphere to the other. In most cases, the connections are between homologous areas and are reciprocal. This is the anatomic structure required for each hemisphere to be kept informed of the activity of the other. These crossing fibers are collectively called a *commissure;* the corpus callosum is the largest (and newest) of the cerebral commissures. (The functional aspects of the corpus callosum are discussed with Fig. 8.)

If the brain is sectioned in the sagittal plane along this interhemispheric fissure, the corpus callosum is divided. This reveals the medial aspect of the brain. Both the frontal and parietal lobes, as well as most of the occipital lobe, are found on the medial aspect of the brain, which is presented in Figure 7.

It is difficult on this view to appreciate the depth of the corpus callosum. In fact, there is a considerable amount of cortical tissue on the medial surface of the hemispheres, as represented by the frontal, parietal, and occipital lobes.

Note on the safe handling of brain tissue: This is a rather old photograph of a brain specimen. Current guidelines recommend the use of disposable gloves when handling any brain tissue, as shown in Figures 3 and 77.

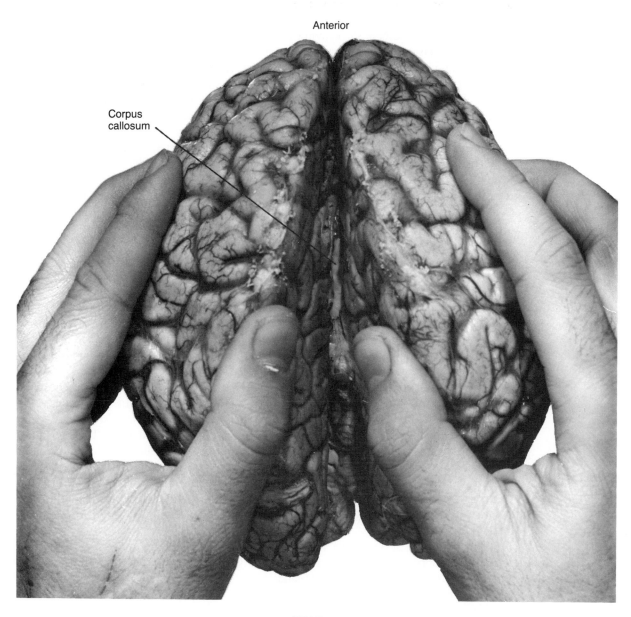

Anterior

Corpus
callosum

FIGURE 6

FIGURE 7   # Medial Aspect of the Brain

The medial view is one of the most important for understanding the gross anatomy of the brain, the brain stem, and the ventricles. The brain has been sectioned in the midline, midsagittally, through the corpus callosum.

The medial aspects of the lobes of the brain are now in view. The central fissure extends onto this part of the brain (although usually not as deep as on the dorsolateral surface). In terms of the sensory and motor homunculi, the leg area of the body is represented on this surface (see Figs. 54 and 57). The medial surface of the frontal lobe is situated anteriorly, with the parietal lobe behind. Moving posteriorly, the parieto-occipital fissure has been opened. The occipital lobe is now visible and is divided by a deep fissure, the *calcarine fissure,* into upper and lower portions. The primary visual area, the area where the visual fibers first arrive in the cerebral cortex, is located along the banks of the calcarine fissure. This area is commonly called area 17 (described with Figs. 56A and 56B). The adjacent areas of the occipital lobe are visual association areas and are known as areas 18 and 19.

Above the corpus callosum is an important gyrus that is part of the limbic system, the *cingulate gyrus* (see Fig. 70). The corpus callosum in this specimen does not have the usual white matter appearance that would be expected. The *septum pellucidum,* a membrane dividing the lateral ventricle of one hemisphere from that of the other side, has been removed, thereby exposing one of the lateral ventricles, which is seen to be situated inferior to the corpus callosum. (The ventricles are described with Figures 10A and 10B.)

This medial view of the brain exposes half of the paired diencephalon (see Figs. 21, 22, and 52). The thalamic portion is found in the middle of the brain, not visible from the outside. A groove, the *hypothalamic sulcus,* divides the thalamus above from the hypothalamic part of the diencephalon below. This sulcus starts at the foramen of Monro (the interventricular foramen; discussed with the ventricles) and ends at the aqueduct of the midbrain. The fiber bundle known as the *fornix,* which is part of the limbic system (see Figs. 70, 71, and 75), courses above the thalamus and is situated just anterior to the interventricular foramen. (In fact, part of this bundle of fibers has been removed from this specimen.) The optic chiasm is found at the anterior aspect of the hypothalamus (see Fig. 5). The *pineal body* (sectioned) is located off the posterior aspect of the diencephalon (see Fig. 22).

The three parts of the brain stem—the *midbrain,* the *pons* (with its bulge anteriorly), and the *medulla* (refer to the ventral view shown in Fig. 21)—can be distinguished on this view. Through the midbrain is a narrow channel for CSF, the *cerebral aqueduct,* also known as the *aqueduct of the midbrain* or the *aqueduct of Sylvius* (see Figs. 10A and 10B). This aqueduct opens into the fourth ventricle, which separates the pons and medulla from the cerebellum. The *fourth ventricle* is said to have a floor, which is the brain stem, and a roof (see Fig. 46); the roof is divided into an upper and lower portion. The upper part consists of a band of white matter known as the *superior medullary velum* (see Figs. 31 and 46). The lower part of the roof of this ventricle is occupied by choroid plexus (see Fig. 27), which has not been preserved on this specimen.

The posterior aspect of the midbrain (behind the aqueduct) is seen to have four "bumps," the *superior and inferior colliculi* (see Fig. 22). The superior colliculi are nuclei associated with vision (see Fig. 56B), and the inferior colliculi are part of the auditory pathway (described with Figs. 39 and 55).

The cerebellum lies behind (or above) the fourth ventricle. It has been sectioned through its midline portion, the *vermis.* Although it is not necessary to name all of the various parts of the vermis, it is useful to know two of them—the *lingula* and the *nodulus.* (The reason for this will become evident when describing the cerebellum [see Fig. 58].) The lingula is that part of the vermis lying immediately above the superior medullary velum. The nodulus is that part of the vermis lying adjacent to the lower portion of the roof of the fourth ventricle.

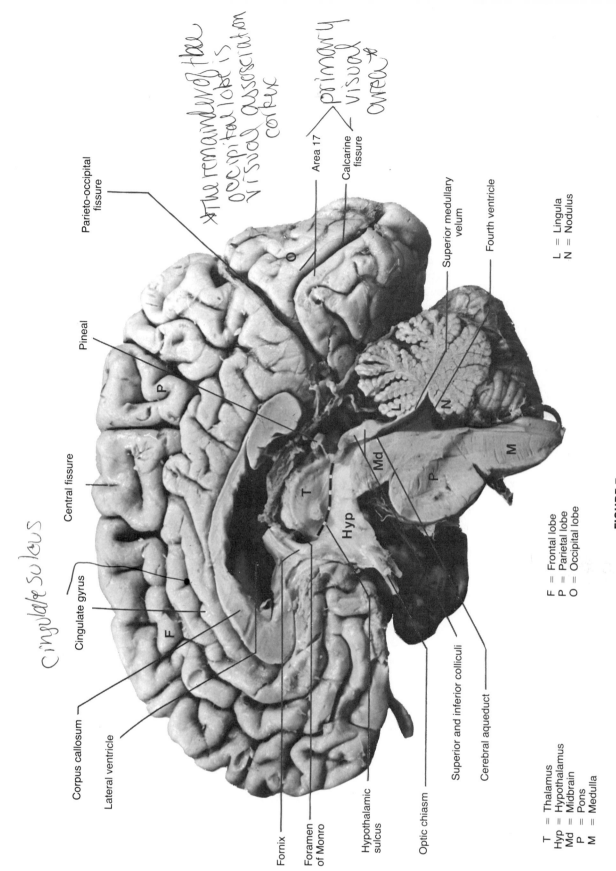

Cingulate sulcus

Central fissure

Cingulate gyrus

Corpus callosum

Lateral ventricle

Fornix

Foramen of Monro

Hypothalamic sulcus

Optic chiasm

Cerebral aqueduct

Superior and inferior colliculi

Parieto-occipital fissure

Pineal

*The remainder of the occipital lobe is visual association cortex

Area 17
Calcarine fissure } primary visual area*

Superior medullary velum

Fourth ventricle

L = Lingula
N = Nodulus

F = Frontal lobe
P = Parietal lobe
O = Occipital lobe

T = Thalamus
Hyp = Hypothalamus
Md = Midbrain
P = Pons
M = Medulla

FIGURE 7

19

FIGURE 8

White Matter: Corpus Callosum

The brain is again seen from the medial view. (Its anterior aspect is on the right side of this photograph.)

The corpus callosum is the massive commissure of the forebrain, connecting homologous regions of the two hemispheres of the cortex across the midline. In a sagittal section, the thickened anterior aspect of the corpus callosum is called the *genu,* and the thickened posterior portion the *splenium* (neither has been labeled).

Cortical tissue has been removed from the specimen, using blunt dissection techniques. The fibers of the corpus callosum can be followed to the cerebral cortex. These fibers intermingle with the other fiber bundles that make up the mass of white matter in the depth of the hemisphere.

In a clinical setting, the corpus callosum is sectioned surgically in certain individuals with intractable epilepsy—that is, epilepsy not controllable with anticonvulsant medication. The idea behind this surgery is to stop the spread of the abnormal discharges from one hemisphere to the other.

Studies done in individuals after surgery have helped to clarify the role of the corpus callosum in normal brain function. Generally, the surgery has been helpful in well-selected cases and there is apparently no noticeable change in the person or in his or her level of brain function. In these individuals, it has been possible to demonstrate under laboratory conditions how the two hemispheres of the brain function independently after sectioning of the corpus callosum. These studies show the consequences of the fact that information is not getting transferred from one hemisphere to the other after the surgery—for example, how the hemispheres respond differently to various stimuli.

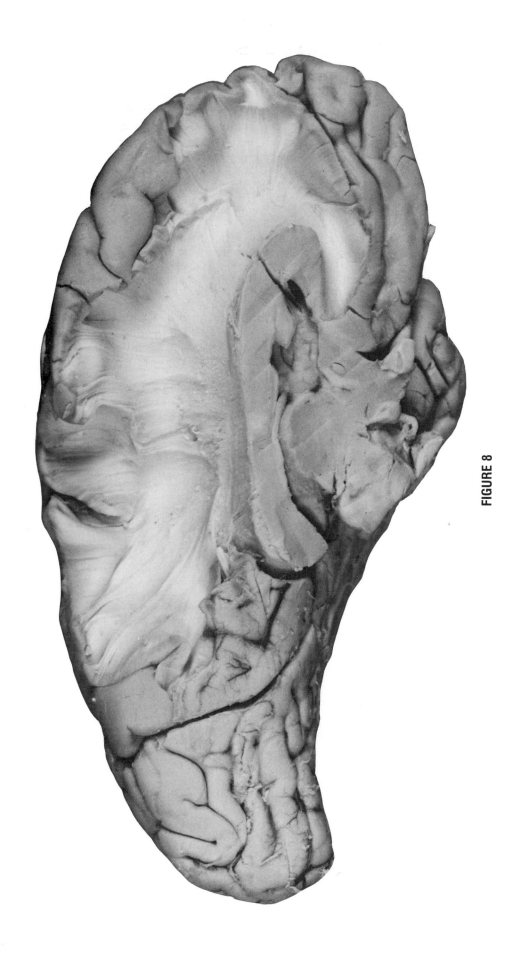

FIGURE 8

FIGURE 9A

White Matter of the Hemispheres

The dorsolateral aspect of the brain is in view in this photograph.

The white matter of the brain has various fiber bundles that can be dissected (with some difficulty) using a blunt instrument (e.g., a wooden tongue depressor). Functionally, some of these are fibers that interconnect different parts of the cerebral cortex on the same side. These are the association bundles.

This specimen has been dissected to show one of the association bundles within the hemispheres. There are also shorter association fibers between adjacent gyri.

These association bundles are extremely important in informing different brain regions of ongoing neuronal processing, thereby allowing for integration of our activities (e.g., sensory with motor and limbic).

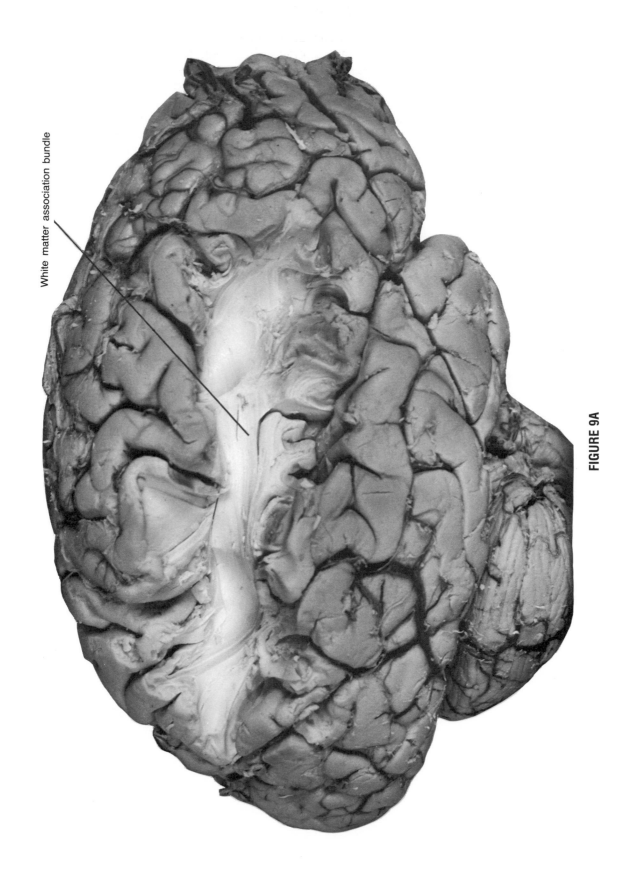

White matter association bundle

FIGURE 9A

FIGURE 9B

White Matter of the Hemispheres: Arcuate Bundle

The *arcuate bundle* is a specific group of association fibers of some importance, particularly on the side dominant for language, which is the left hemisphere in most people. This fiber bundle connects the two cortical areas for language (see Fig. 2), Broca's area anteriorly with Wernicke's area posteriorly.

Damage to these fibers in humans causes a disruption of language, called *conduction aphasia*. *Aphasia* is a general term for a disruption or disorder of language. In conduction aphasia, the person has normal comprehension (intact Wernicke's area) and fluent speech (intact Broca's area). The only deficit is an inability to repeat what has been heard. This is usually tested by asking the patient to repeat single words or phrases whose meaning cannot be readily understood (e.g., the phrase "no ifs, ands, or buts").

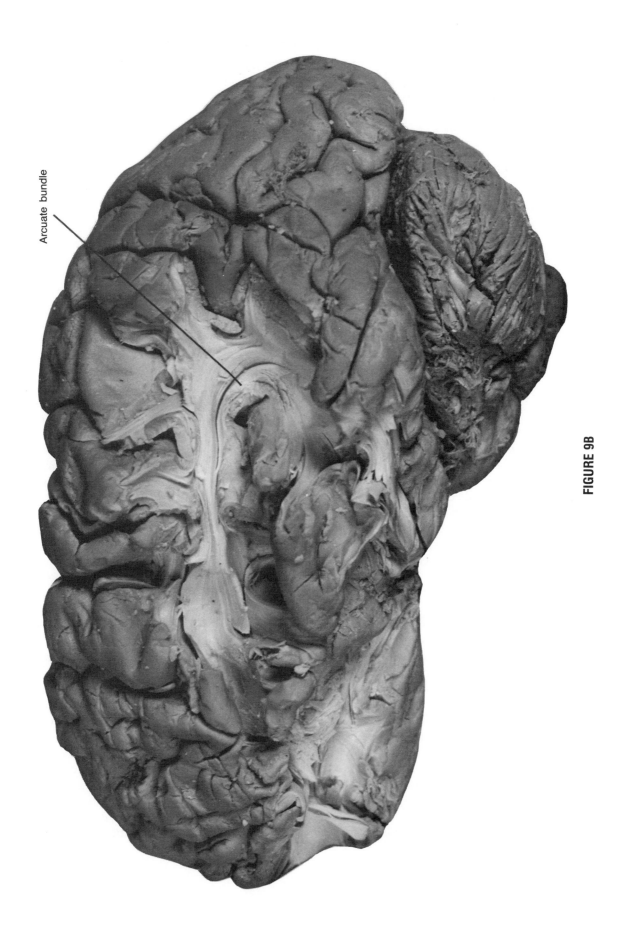

Arcuate bundle

FIGURE 9B

25

PART A-II

INTERNAL STRUCTURES: VENTRICLES, BASAL GANGLIA, AND INTERNAL CAPSULE
(Figures 10–19)

FIGURE 10A   Ventricles: Lateral View

The ventricles of the brain are what remain of the original neural tube, the tube that was present during development. The cells of the nervous system, both neurons and glia, originated from a germinal matrix that was located adjacent to the lining of this tube. As the nervous system develops, the mass of tissue grows and the size of the tube diminishes in proportion. The ventricles are filled with CSF.

The parts of the tube that remain in the hemispheres are called the *cerebral ventricles,* also called the *lateral ventricles.* The lateral ventricle of one hemisphere is shown from the lateral perspective. It is shaped like the letter C in reverse; it curves posteriorly to enter into the temporal lobe. The ventricle has various parts—the *frontal* (anterior) *horn,* which lies deep within the frontal lobes; the central portion or *body,* which lies deep within the parietal lobes; and the *inferior horn,* which goes into the temporal lobes. In addition, there may be an extension into the occipital lobes, called the *occipital* or *posterior horn.* These lateral ventricles are also called ventricles I and II (assigned arbitrarily).

Each lateral ventricle is connected to the midline *third ventricle* by the *foramen of Monro* (*interventricular foramen*). The third ventricle could also be called the *ventricle of the diencephalon* (see also Fig. 22). The system then narrows considerably through the midbrain and is now called the *aqueduct of the midbrain, the cerebral aqueduct,* or the *aqueduct of Sylvius* (see Fig. 7). In the hindbrain region—the area consisting of pons, medulla, and cerebellum—it widens again to form the *fourth ventricle* (see Fig. 46). The channel continues within the CNS and becomes the very narrow *central canal* of the spinal cord.

Within the ventricles is specialized tissue, the *choroid plexus.* It is made up of the lining cells of the ventricles, called the *ependyma,* and pia with blood vessels (see Fig. 11). The choroid plexus is the tissue responsible for the formation of most of the CSF. It is found in the body and inferior horn of the lateral ventricle, in the roof of the third ventricle, and in the lower half of the roof of the fourth ventricle. The tissue forms large invaginations into the ventricles in each of these locations (unfortunately, none of these are visible in the photographic views).

CSF flows through the ventricular system, from the lateral ventricles, through the interventricular foramina into the third ventricle, then through the narrow aqueduct and into the fourth ventricle. At the bottom of the fourth ventricle, CSF exits from the ventricular system and enters the subarachnoid space.

The exit points are foramina in the fourth ventricle. The major exit is the *foramen of Magendie,* in the midline. There are two additional exits of the CSF laterally from the fourth ventricle; these are the *foramina of Luschka* and will be seen in another perspective (see Fig. 10B). The CSF then enters one of the enlargements of the subarachnoid space, called a *cistern;* this particular one is called the *cisterna magna,* the *cerebellomedullary cistern.* It lies below the cerebellum and is found inside the skull, just above the foramen magnum.

CSF flows through the subarachnoid space (shown diagrammatically in Fig. 11). It is reabsorbed back into the venous system through the arachnoid villi, which are protrusions of the arachnoid into the venous dural sinuses. These can be seen as collections of villi on the intact brain, called *arachnoid granulations* (see Fig. 1; shown diagrammatically in Fig. 11).

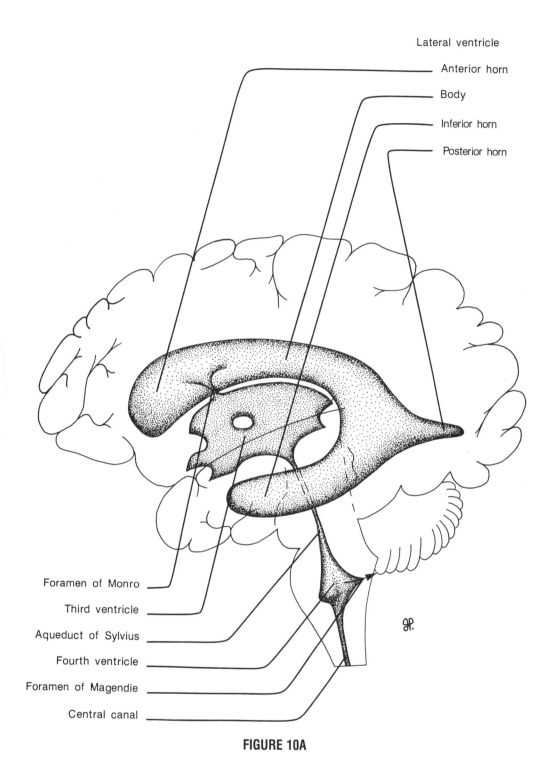

Lateral ventricle

Anterior horn

Body

Inferior horn

Posterior horn

Foramen of Monro

Third ventricle

Aqueduct of Sylvius

Fourth ventricle

Foramen of Magendie

Central canal

FIGURE 10A

FIGURE 10B   # Ventricles: Anterior View

In the anterior view, one can see both lateral ventricles and the short interventricular foramina on both sides, connecting each lateral ventricle with the midline third ventricle. The diencephalon is found on either side of the third ventricle (see Fig. 22).

After flowing through the aqueduct of the midbrain, CSF enters the fourth ventricle, which also straddles the midline. The fourth ventricle is diamond shaped, and the lateral recesses carry CSF into the cisterna magna through the foramina of Luschka, the lateral apertures, one on each side.

The flow of CSF can be interrupted or blocked at various key points. One of the most common is the cerebral aqueduct, the aqueduct of the midbrain. Since a considerable amount of CSF is formed upstream in the lateral (and third) ventricles, this creates a damming effect. This causes a marked enlargement of the ventricles, which can be seen with imaging techniques (e.g., computed tomography [CT] scan). The CSF flow can be blocked developmentally, following a meningitis, by a tumor in the region, or for a variety of other reasons. The end result is called *hydrocephalus*.

Hydrocephalus in the infant stage occurs, often spontaneously, for unknown reasons. Because the sutures of the infant's skull are not yet fused, it leads to an enlargement of the head. Clinical assessment of infants includes measuring the size of the head and charting this in the same way as one charts height and weight. Clinical treatment of this condition, after evaluation of the causative factor, includes shunting the CSF out of the ventricles into one of the body cavities. Untreated hydrocephalus will eventually lead to a compression of the nervous tissue of the hemispheres and to damage to this developing tissue.

In adults, hydrocephalus caused by a blockage of the CSF flow leads to an increase in intracranial pressure. The cause is usually a tumor, and in addition to the specific symptoms, the patient will complain of headache. Clinical evaluation involves the neurologist and usually the neuroradiologist, using a variety of imaging techniques.

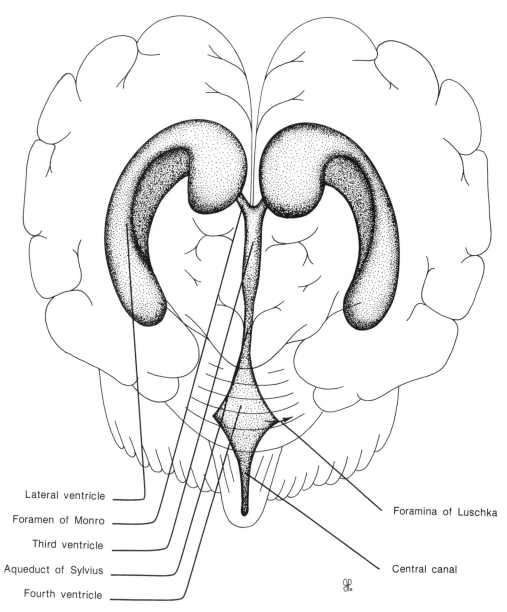

Lateral ventricle

Foramen of Monro

Third ventricle

Aqueduct of Sylvius

Fourth ventricle

Foramina of Luschka

Central canal

FIGURE 10B

FIGURE 11   # Cerebrospinal Fluid

This is a schematic representation of the relationship between the brain tissue, CSF, and the cerebral blood vessels. CSF is found in the ventricles and in the subarachnoid space; the flow of CSF is shown. The physiologic barriers between the various compartments are also indicated.

The ventricles of the brain are lined with a layer of cells known as the *ependyma*. In certain loci within each of the ventricles, the ependymal cells and the pia meet, forming the *choroid plexus,* which invaginates into the ventricle. Functionally, the choroid plexus has a vascular layer (i.e., the pia) on the inside and the ependymal layer on the ventricular side. CSF is actively secreted by the choroid plexus. There is a physical barrier between the blood vessels on the inside of the choroid plexus and the ventricle, the blood–CSF barrier (B-CSF-B in the diagram). The ionic composition of CSF is different from that of serum.

CSF leaves the ventricular system from the fourth ventricle, as indicated schematically in the diagram. In the intact brain, this occurs via the medially placed foramen of Magendie and the two laterally placed foramina of Luschka (see Figs. 10A and 10B). CSF flows through the *subarachnoid space* (SAS) and is returned to the venous system. The return is through the arachnoid villi, which protrude into the venous sinuses of the brain, particularly the superior sagittal sinus (see Fig. 1).

There is no real barrier between the intercellular tissue of the brain and the CSF, through either the ependyma or the pia. This is depicted by the arrows, which indicate a free communication between these compartments. Therefore, substances found in detectable amounts in the intercellular spaces of the brain may be found in the CSF.

On the other hand, there is a real barrier, both structural and functional, between the blood vessels and the brain tissue. This is called the blood–brain barrier (BBB) and is situated at the level of the brain capillaries. Only oxygen, carbon dioxide, glucose, and other small molecules are normally able to cross the blood–brain barrier.

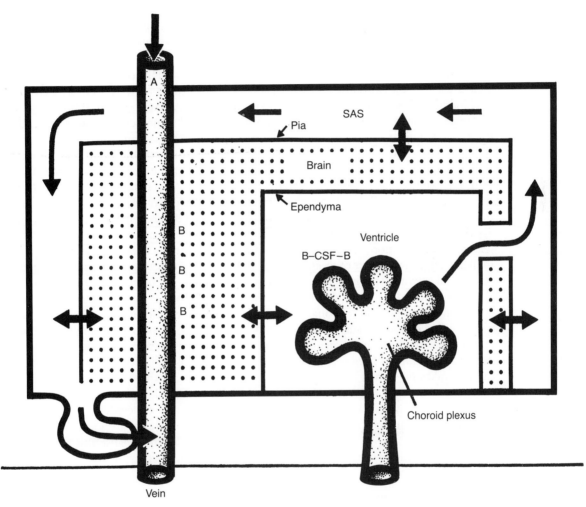

BBB = Blood–brain barrier   B–CSF–B = Blood–CSF barrier
A = Artery   SAS = Subarachnoid space

FIGURE 11

FIGURE 12   # Basal Ganglia I (Orientation)

The basal ganglia are large collections of neurons belonging embryologically to the forebrain and the diencephalon. Our ideas about what the basal ganglia do are partially based on the anatomy of the system (i.e., its connections), and partially derived from disease states affecting these neurons. In general, humans with lesions in the basal ganglia have some form of motor dysfunction—that is, a movement disorder.

From the strictly anatomic point of view, the basal ganglia are collections of neurons within the hemispheres. Traditionally, these would include the *caudate nucleus,* the *putamen,* the *globus pallidus,* and the *amygdala.* From the functional point of view and based on the complex pattern of interconnections, two other nuclei should be included with the description of the basal ganglia—the *subthalamic nucleus* (part of the diencephalon) and the *substantia nigra* (located in the midbrain). Based on similar arguments, the amygdala is no longer considered a part of the basal ganglia.

Overall, the basal ganglia receive much of their input from the cortex, the motor areas as well as wide areas of association cortex. There are intricate connections between the various parts of the system (involving different neurotransmitters), and the output is directed via the thalamus mainly to premotor, supplementary motor, and frontal cortical areas. Therefore, the basal ganglia act as a subloop of the motor system by altering cortical activity (see Fig. 57).

This large group of neurons is thought to be involved in the control of complex patterns of motor activity, such as skilled movements (e.g., writing). There are two aspects to this involvement. The first concerns the initiation of the movement. The second concerns the quality of the performance of the motor task. It seems that different parts of the basal ganglia are concerned with how rapidly a movement is to be performed and the magnitude of the movement. In addition, some of the structures that make up the basal ganglia are thought to influence cognitive aspects of motor control, helping to plan the sequence of tasks needed for purposeful activity. This is sometimes referred to as as the *selection of motor strategies*.

The functional role of this large collection of neurons is best illustrated by clinical conditions affecting this neuronal system. These disease entities include abnormal movements, called *dyskinesias,* such as *chorea* (jerky movements), *athetosis* (writhing movements), and *tremors* (rhythmic movements). The most common condition affecting this group of neurons is *Parkinson's disease.* A person with this disease has difficulty initiating movements, the face takes on a masklike appearance with loss of facial expressiveness, and he or she experiences muscular rigidity, a slowing of movements (bradykinesia), and a tremor of the hands at rest that goes away with purposeful movements (and in sleep).

The basal ganglia, from the point of view of strict anatomy, are located within the cerebral hemispheres. In fact, the term *ganglia* is inappropriate because this term usually applies to collections of neurons in the peripheral nervous system; hence they should be thought of as *nuclei.*

- The *caudate nucleus* has three portions:
    - The head, located within the frontal lobe
    - The body, located deep in the parietal lobe
    - The tail, which goes into the temporal lobe
- The *lentiform nucleus* is so named because it is lens shaped. In fact, it is composed of two nuclei (see Fig. 16)—the putamen and the globus pallidus. It is situated laterally and is found deep in the hemispheres within the central white matter.

Both the caudate nucleus and the lentiform nucleus are found below the level of the corpus callosum.

By definition, the *amygdala* (not shown) is a part of the basal ganglia. It is a group of neurons located within the hemisphere. Because most of its connections and functions are with the limbic system, our "emotional brain," discussion of this nucleus is usually deferred to that time (see Section G, Fig. 72). Diseases of the basal ganglia often have an emotional component. As we will see later (see Fig. 82A), the ventral parts of the lentiform nucleus may be a functional part of the limbic system.

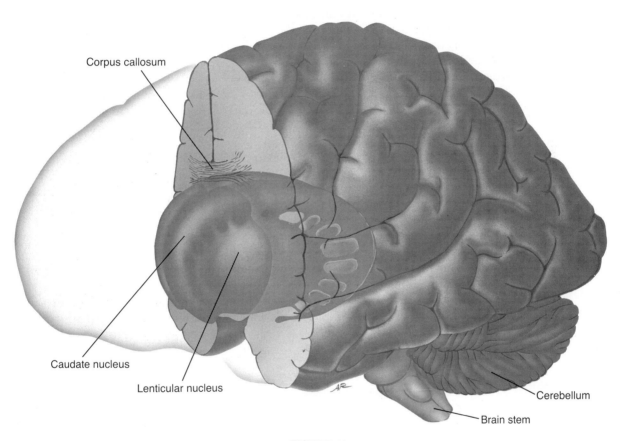

Corpus callosum

Caudate nucleus

Lenticular nucleus

Cerebellum

Brain stem

FIGURE 12

33

FIGURE 13 # Basal Ganglia and Ventricles

The basal ganglia are being visualized deep in the hemisphere, from the lateral perspective. The various parts include the caudate nucleus, the lentiform nucleus (and sometimes also the amygdala). Included in this view is the ventricular system (as in Fig. 10A) and the thalamus, which lies adjacent to the third ventricle (see Fig. 22).

All three parts of the caudate nucleus—the head, body, and tail—are situated adjacent to the lateral ventricle. In fact, the head protrudes into the anterior horn of the lateral ventricle (see Fig. 18). The body of the caudate lies adjacent to the body of the ventricle (see Figs. 19 and 55), with the tail following the ventricle into the temporal lobe (see Figs. 55 and 76).

The lentiform nucleus is made up of two distinct parts, the *putamen* and the *globus pallidus*. These are different functional parts of the basal ganglia that are found together, forming a lens-shaped nucleus called the *lentiform nucleus*. The lens configuration can easily be seen in a horizontal section through the hemispheres (see Fig. 18).

In this view, one can see the connection between the caudate and the lentiform nuclei. Specifically, this is the connection between the caudate and putamen; these are in fact the same neurons from an embryologic point of view. As fiber systems develop, these nuclei become separated from each other by the anterior limb of the internal capsule (see Figs. 16 through 18). Some connecting strands of tissue can still be found in the adult brain on a few horizontal sections through the lowermost parts of these nuclei. (These connecting strands will be shown in subsequent diagrams.)

The other nucleus shown in this diagram is the *thalamus*, part of the diencephalon. Although the diencephalon belongs to another region and will be discussed later (see Figs. 21 and 22, and Section D), it is also located in the depths of the hemispheres, on either side of the third ventricle. Therefore, any section in the horizontal plane at the appropriate level includes cuts through the thalamus.

A horizontal section through the brain at the level of the lateral fissure would reveal all these structures (see Fig. 18). The internal capsule, which consists of a collection of fibers (described in Fig. 17), is situated between the lentiform nucleus, the head of the caudate, and the thalamus.

As mentioned, although the amygdala (the amygdaloid nucleus) is by definition part of the basal ganglia, its connections are with the limbic system, and a discussion of this nucleus will be deferred until then (see Fig. 72).

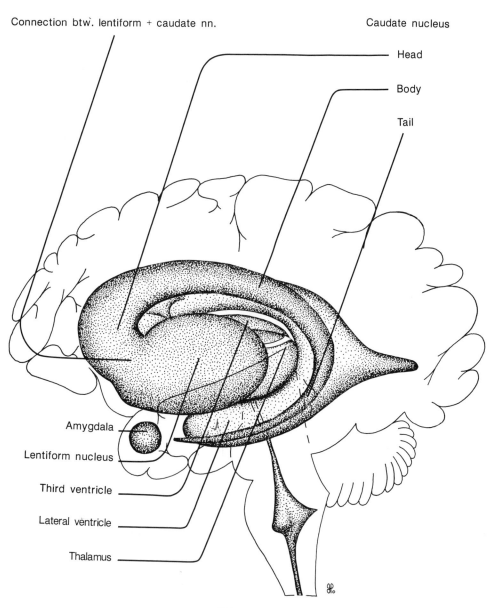

Connection btw. lentiform + caudate nn.

Caudate nucleus

Head

Body

Tail

Amygdala

Lentiform nucleus

Third ventricle

Lateral ventricle

Thalamus

FIGURE 13

FIGURE 14 # Basal Ganglia II

The basal ganglia are seen in isolation from the lateral perspective as well as from above, allowing a view of the caudate nucleus of both sides.

The various parts of the caudate nucleus are easily recognized—head, body, and tail. The tail follows the inferior horn of the lateral ventricle into the temporal lobe (see Figs. 12, 13, and 76). In a coronal section (see Figs. 19 and 78), the tail of the caudate is found above the inferior horn of the lateral ventricle.

Lentiform nucleus (also called the lenticular nucleus) is only a descriptive name that means lens shaped. This shape is seen on a horizontal section of the hemispheres (see Fig. 18) at the level of this nucleus. The nucleus is in fact composed of two distinct parts—the putamen laterally and the globus pallidus medially. When viewing the basal ganglia from the lateral perspective, one sees only the putamen part.

Strands of tissue are seen connecting the caudate nucleus with the lentiform nucleus; in fact, they connect the caudate with the putamen (as discussed with Fig. 13). The caudate and the putamen are collectively called the *neostriatum,* or simply the *striatum.*

The inferior portions of the putamen and globus pallidus are found at the level of the *anterior commissure.* It is this lower part of the lentiform nucleus that may have a limbic connection (see Fig. 82A). The anterior commissure connects the amygdala and other temporal lobe structures of the two sides (discussed further with Fig. 70).

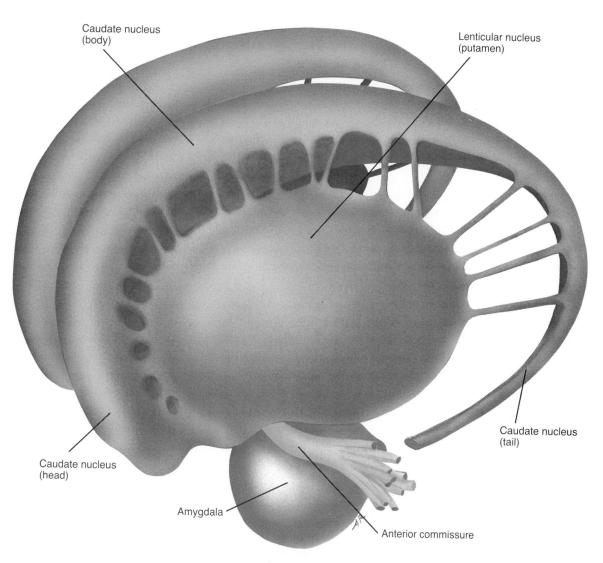

Caudate nucleus
(body)

Lenticular nucleus
(putamen)

Caudate nucleus
(tail)

Caudate nucleus
(head)

Amygdala

Anterior commissure

FIGURE 14

FIGURE 15   # Basal Ganglia III

This view has been obtained by removing all parts of the basal ganglia of one hemisphere, except the tail of the caudate and the amygdala. This exposes the lentiform nucleus of the "distal" side; the lentiform nucleus is thus being visualized from a medial perspective. This nucleus is now seen to be composed of its two portions, the putamen laterally and the globus pallidus, which is medially placed (see also Fig. 16).

The globus pallidus itself is composed of two segments, the *medial* and *lateral segments,* also known as internal and external segments, respectively. (These can also be seen in the horizontal section of the brain in Figure 18.) This subdivision of the globus pallidus is important functionally.

Strands of cells are seen connecting the various portions of the caudate with the putamen. As has been explained previously, the caudate and putamen are in fact the same neurons embryologically. Together they are known as the *neostriatum* (in some texts, they are simply called the *striatum*). This nuclear structure has been separated into two components by groups of axons, which collectively are called the *internal capsule* (see Fig. 17). These fiber bundles "fill the spaces" between the cellular strands.

The illustration also includes the two other parts of the functional basal ganglia—the subthalamic nucleus and the substantia nigra.

■ The *subthalamic region* is situated below the level of the diencephalon. The small nucleus in this area is connected with the globus pallidus, both receiving fibers from and sending fibers to different parts of that nucleus.

Clinically, the motor abnormality associated with a lesion of the subthalamic nucleus is called *hemiballismus*. The sufferer (human or animal) experiences sudden flinging movements of one or both limbs, on the opposite side of the body from the lesioned nucleus.

■ The substantia nigra is located in the midbrain region as an elongated nucleus (see Fig. 54). It is composed of two parts (see Figs. 28 and 29):
   ■ The *pars reticulata* is situated more ventrally.
      It receives fibers from the basal ganglia and is involved in the output from the basal ganglia.
   ■ The *pars compacta* has the pigment-containing cells.
      These neurons project their fibers to the putamen.
      The neurotransmitter involved is dopamine.

It is the degeneration of these dopamine-containing neurons, with the consequent loss of their dopamine input to the basal ganglia, that leads to the clinical entity of *Parkinson's disease*.

Information flows into the caudate and putamen from all areas of the cerebral cortex (in a topographic manner), from the substantia nigra (pars compacta), and from the centromedian nucleus of the thalamus (see Figs. 53 and 57). This information is processed and passed on to the globus pallidus (and the pars reticulata of the substantia nigra of the midbrain). The most important output from the basal ganglia is from the inner segment of the globus pallidus. Most of this information is relayed to the thalamus, and from specific relay nuclei to the prefrontal and premotor cortical areas (see Fig. 57). These are the cortical areas concerned with motor planning and motor control.

The *nucleus accumbens* is somewhat unique in that it seems to consist of a mix of neurons from the basal ganglia and from the limbic structures in the region. The functional role of this nucleus has not yet been fully elucidated (discussed with Fig. 82A).

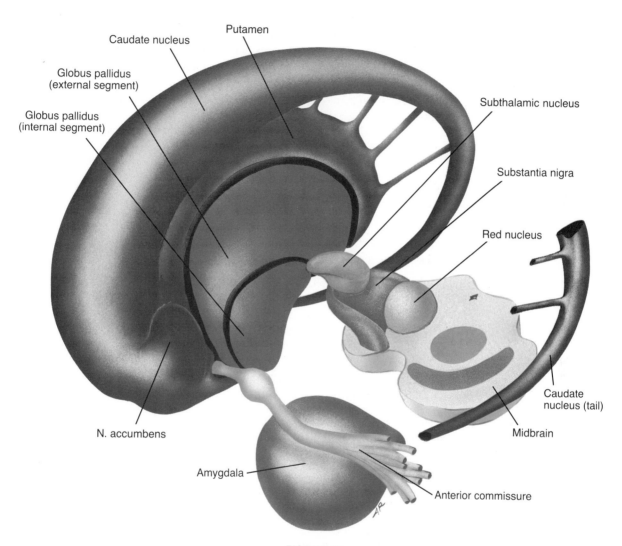

Caudate nucleus

Putamen

Globus pallidus
(external segment)

Globus pallidus
(internal segment)

Subthalamic nucleus

Substantia nigra

Red nucleus

Caudate
nucleus (tail)

N. accumbens

Midbrain

Amygdala

Anterior commissure

FIGURE 15

FIGURE 16   # Basal Ganglia IV

Removal of the head of the caudate nucleus (and some of its body) exposes the putamen more completely. The area between the two nuclei is now revealed. In the brain, this area is filled in with axons, which will be discussed with the next diagram.

Many years ago, it was common to refer to the basal ganglia as part of the *extrapyramidal* motor system (in contrast to the *pyramidal* motor system; discussed with Fig. 41, the corticospinal tract). It is now known that the basal ganglia exert their influence through the appropriate parts of the cerebral cortex, which then act either directly (i.e., using the corticospinal [pyramidal] tract) or indirectly (via certain brain stem nuclei) to alter motor activity. The term *extrapyramidal* should probably be abandoned but is still frequently encountered in a clinical setting. Other terms could be used, such as *nonpyramidal* or simply *basal ganglia*. At best, one could perhaps consider this system in the same way as one is accustomed to viewing the influence of the cerebellum on motor control (see Section E).

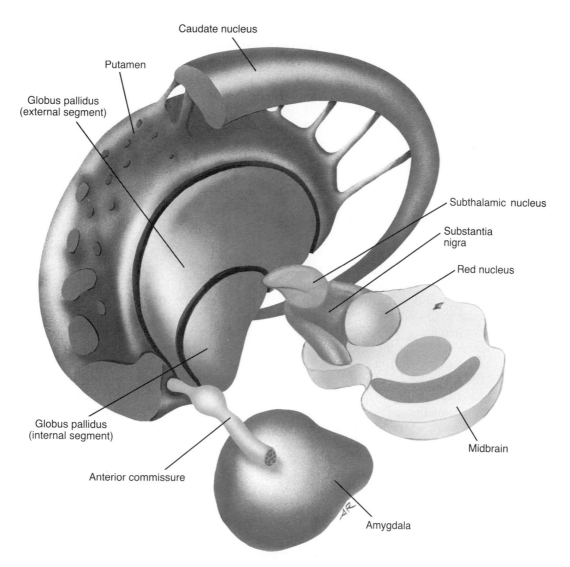

Caudate nucleus

Putamen

Globus pallidus
(external segment)

Subthalamic nucleus

Substantia
nigra

Red nucleus

Globus pallidus
(internal segment)

Anterior commissure

Midbrain

Amygdala

FIGURE 16

41

FIGURE 17   # Internal Capsule

As noted earlier, a group of fibers has separated off the two parts of the neostriatum from each other, the caudate from the putamen. This fiber system carries axons that are coming down from the cortex, and these form part of the *internal capsule—its anterior limb.*

Situated medially at the level of the lentiform nucleus is the *thalamus,* which is part of the diencephalon (see Section D). It is a paired nuclear structure that is located on both sides of the third ventricle (see Figs. 22 and 52). The fiber system that runs between the thalamus (medially) and the lentiform nucleus (laterally) is the *posterior limb* of the internal capsule.

The posterior limb carries most of the descending fibers to the brain stem (cortico-bulbar; see Fig. 40) and spinal cord (corticospinal; see Fig. 41). The somatosensory fibers from the body and face, after synapsing in the thalamus, reach the cortex by traveling in the posterior limb (see Fig. 54).

In addition, some axons from the cortex are destined for the cerebellum, after synapsing first in the pontine nuclei (see Fig. 59). These corticopontine fibers descend in both the anterior and posterior limbs of the internal capsule.

The segregation of the various fibers occurs in the *cerebral peduncle* of the *midbrain,* where the corticopontine fibers are found in the outer and inner thirds of the peduncle, and the corticobulbar and corticospinal fibers are located in the middle third (see Figs. 40 and 48).

Other fiber systems emanating from the thalamus are often described in relation to the internal capsule. For example, the visual radiation is situated posterior to the internal capsule, yet functionally is part of it (see Figs. 56A and 56B). The same is true of the auditory radiation, which runs inferiorly (see Fig. 55).

The internal capsule can also be seen in a horizontal section of the brain (see Fig. 18). In this view, the internal capsule (of each side) is seen to be V shaped. The anterior portion between the caudate and lentiform nuclei is the anterior limb. The portion between the lentiform nucleus and the thalamus is the posterior limb. The bend of the V is called the *genu,* and it is situated medially.

In summary, at the level of the internal capsule are the ascending fibers from thalamus to cortex, as well as the descending fibers from widespread areas of the cerebral cortex to the thalamus and the rest of the neuraxis. These ascending and descending fibers are also called *projection fibers* (discussed in the Introduction to Section A). This whole fiber system is sometimes likened to a funnel, with the top of the funnel being the cerebral cortex and the stem being the cerebral peduncle. The base of the funnel would be the internal capsule. The main point is that the various fiber systems, both ascending and descending, are condensed together in the region of the internal capsule.

The area of the internal capsule is clinically important because of the frequency of lesions here. The blood vessels that supply the internal capsule come from the middle cerebral artery as it courses in the lateral fissure; they are known as the *striate arteries* (see Fig. 82A). For reasons not clearly understood, these blood vessels are prone to rupture. This type of pathologic event destroys the surrounding axons. Because of the high packing density of the axons in this region, a small lesion can create extensive disruption of descending and ascending pathways. This is the underlying neuroanatomy of one of the most common types of "stroke" seen clinically. An unfortunate frequent consequence of this lesion is paralysis on one side of the body that is often permanent.

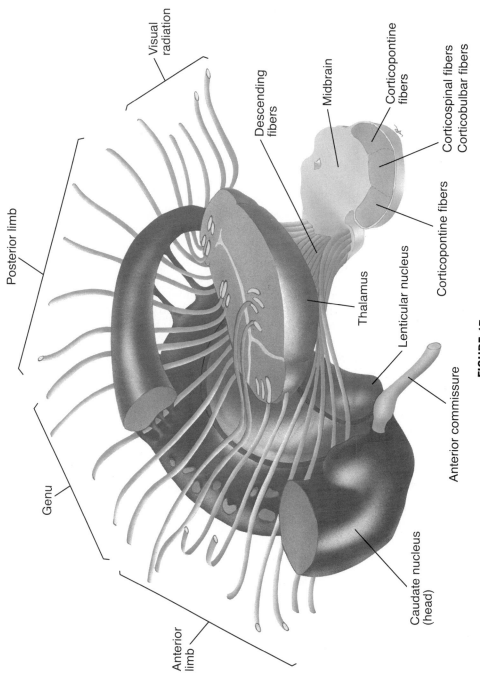

Visual radiation

Posterior limb

Genu

Anterior limb

Descending fibers

Midbrain

Corticopontine fibers

Corticospinal fibers
Corticobulbar fibers

Corticopontine fibers

Thalamus

Lenticular nucleus

Anterior commissure

Caudate nucleus (head)

FIGURE 17

43

FIGURE 18

Horizontal Section of the Hemispheres (Photographic View)

The brain has been sectioned in the horizontal plane at the level of the lateral fissure. This view exposes the white matter of the hemispheres and the basal ganglia. A view similar to this is commonly presented in brain scans of patients. Understanding the topography of the structures seen in this view will be of immeasurable importance once the student enters the clinical setting.

The basal ganglia are present when the brain is sectioned at this level. The head of the caudate nucleus is seen protruding into the lateral ventricle. The lentiform nucleus is shaped somewhat like a lens and is demarcated by white matter. The outer portion of the lentiform nucleus is darker and the inner portion is lighter because of the presence of more fibers within the latter part. The outer part is the putamen, and the inner portion is the globus pallidus. Depending on the level of the section, it is sometimes possible (as in the right side of the photograph) to see the two subdivisions of the globus pallidus, the internal and external segments (see Figs. 15 and 16).

The white matter medial to the lentiform nucleus is the *internal capsule*. It is divisible into an anterior portion, the *anterior limb,* and a *posterior limb;* the base of the V is known as the *genu.* The anterior limb separates the lentiform nucleus from the head of the caudate nucleus. This portion of the caudate nucleus is related to the anterior horn of the lateral ventricle, which is cut through its lowermost part and is represented in this photograph by a very small cavity. Some strands of gray matter located within the anterior limb represent the tissue that unites the caudate nucleus with the putamen (as shown in Fig. 14). The posterior limb of the internal capsule separates the lentiform nucleus from the thalamus. (This relationship can be further understood by examining Figure 17.)

Lateral to the lentiform nucleus is another thin strip of tissue, the *claustrum,* whose functional contribution is not known. Lateral to this is the cortex of the insula. Posteriorly, behind the thalamus, the cerebellum is visible.

It is also possible to see another portion of the lateral ventricle deep within the parietal lobe. The ventricle is sectioned at this level as it enters into the temporal lobe and is becoming the inferior horn of the lateral ventricle (see Fig. 10A).

Anterior

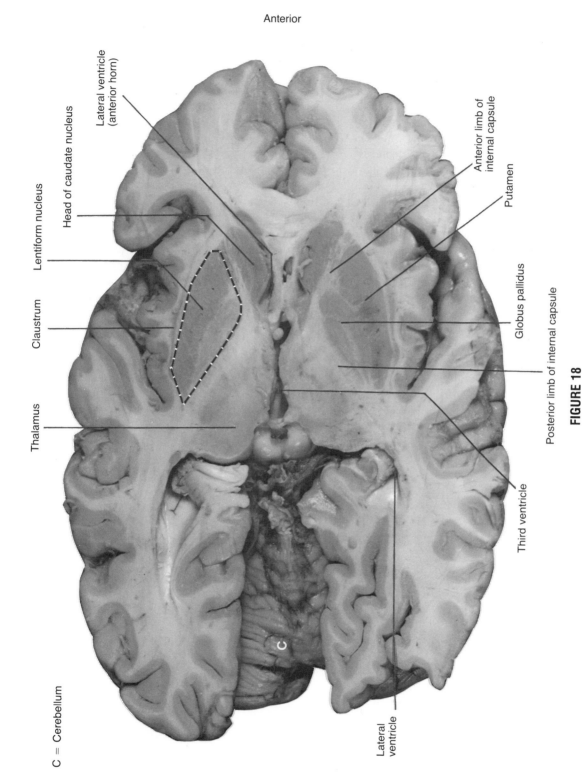

Lateral ventricle
(anterior horn)

Head of caudate nucleus

Lentiform nucleus

Claustrum

Thalamus

Anterior limb of
internal capsule

Putamen

Globus pallidus

Posterior limb of internal capsule

Third ventricle

Lateral
ventricle

C = Cerebellum

FIGURE 18

45

FIGURE 19

Coronal Section: Hemispheres and Internal Capsule (Photographic View)

This is another view of the internal aspect of the hemispheres. The brain is sectioned in the coronal (frontal) plane through the diencephalic region. This particular section has only a small part of the cavity of the third ventricle present in the midline, separating the thalamus of one side from that of the other (see Fig. 22).

The fibers of the corpus callosum are seen crossing the midline at the bottom of the interhemispheric fissure (see Fig. 6). Below the corpus callosum are the two cavities of the lateral ventricle, represented at this plane by the body of the ventricles. At the outer margins of the ventricle is a dark nuclear structure, the body of the caudate nucleus. Below the ventricle is the thalamus. The fornix (see Figs. 70, 71, and 72; explained with Figs. 75 and 76) is also seen as it courses over the thalamus.

Lateral to the thalamus is the posterior limb of the internal capsule. More laterally is the lentiform nucleus; because the brain has not been sectioned symmetrically, more of this nucleus is found on the left side of the photograph.

Separating the parietal lobe (above) from the temporal lobe (below) is the lateral fissure, in the depths of which is the insula (see Fig. 3). A section at the level of the lateral fissure passes through the lentiform nucleus and the thalamus, giving the picture seen in Figure 18.

Because the section was not cut symmetrically, the inferior horn of the lateral ventricle is found only on the right side of this photograph, in the temporal lobe (see also Fig. 78).

On both this photograph and Figure 18, the cerebral cortex is seen on the external aspect of the hemisphere as the gray matter, with the white matter visible internally. It is not possible to separate out the various fiber systems of the white matter in this photographic view.

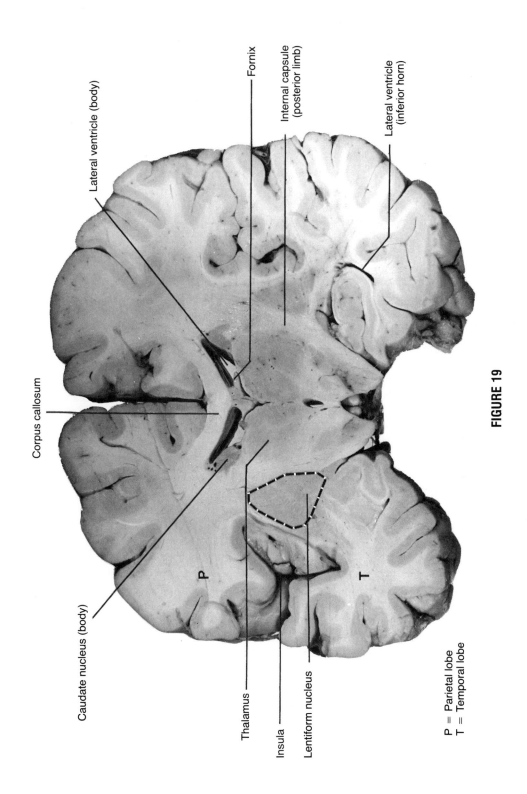

Lateral ventricle (body)

Fornix

Internal capsule (posterior limb)

Lateral ventricle (inferior horn)

Corpus callosum

Caudate nucleus (body)

Thalamus

Insula

Lentiform nucleus

P = Parietal lobe
T = Temporal lobe

P

T

FIGURE 19

PART A-III

BLOOD SUPPLY

FIGURE 20

Arterial Circle of Willis (Photographic View)

The arterial circle of Willis is formed by the vertebral and common carotid arteries. It lies at the base of the brain, surrounding the optic chiasm and the hypothalamus. Within the skull, it is situated above the pituitary fossa (and gland). This exposure of the arterial circle of Willis has been accomplished by excising most of the optic chiasm.

The cut end of the *internal carotid artery* is seen more clearly on the left side. This artery divides into the *middle cerebral artery* and the *anterior cerebral artery*. The middle cerebral artery courses within the lateral fissure. By removing the optic chiasm, the anterior cerebral arteries can be followed anteriorly. Where they meet would be found an extremely short artery connecting the two of them, the *anterior communicating artery*.

The vertebrobasilar system was described with Figure 4 (it supplies the brain stem and cerebellum). The *basilar artery* terminates by dividing into two *posterior cerebral arteries*. Each connects, via the *posterior communicating artery* (one on each side), with the internal carotid (or middle cerebral) artery. This specimen has been selected because the posterior communicating arteries are larger than usual and so could be shown clearly on this photograph. (They can also be seen in Figure 4, although there they are not labeled and are much smaller.)

Therefore, the arterial circle of Willis encircles the optic chiasm, the pituitary stalk, and the mammillary nuclei of the hypothalamus (see Fig. 5). Small arteries from the circle provide the blood supply to the diencephalon and to portions of the internal capsule and basal ganglia.

One of the most important branches of the middle cerebral artery within the lateral fissure is the group of arteries that supply the remainder of the internal capsule and the basal ganglia. These are known as the *striate arteries* (see Figs. 82A and 82B; discussed also with Fig. 17). These small arteries (not shown here) penetrate the brain at the posterior end of the olfactory tract (see Fig. 4).

Branches of the arterial circle supply the hemispheres. The anterior cerebral artery perfuses the medial aspects of the hemispheres, above the corpus callosum (see Fig. 7). The middle cerebral artery emerges from the lateral fissure to supply almost all of the dorsolateral portions of the hemispheres (see Fig. 2). The posterior cerebral arteries provide the blood supply to the inferior parts of the temporal lobe and to the occipital lobe (see Figs. 4 and 5), including the primary visual area. Where the territories overlap, there is a region, known as the *watershed zone,* where the blood supply may be marginally adequate.

Involvement of a particular branch of an artery, either by occlusion or by hemorrhage, disrupts the blood supply to a specific area of the brain. Disruption of the blood supply results in a loss of function, which reflects the functional contribution of that part of the brain. In some people, the communicating branches of the circle of Willis may be large enough to shunt blood from one branch or one side to another. Visualization of the arterial (and venous) branches is done by injecting a radiopaque substance into the arteries (this procedure is done by a neuroradiologist) and following its course by a rapid series of roentgenograms (called an *arteriogram*). Brain hemorrhage and infarction can now be visualized by CT scanning.

One of the characteristic vascular lesions in the vessels forming the arterial circle of Willis is a *berry aneurysm.* This is caused by a weakness of part of the wall of the artery, which results in a local ballooning of the artery. Often, berry aneurysms rupture spontaneously, particularly if there is accompanying hypertension. This sudden rupture occurs into the subarachnoid space and may also involve nervous tissue of the base of the brain. The whole event is known as a *subarachnoid hemorrhage* and must be considered when one is faced clinically with a major cerebrovascular accident.

Anterior

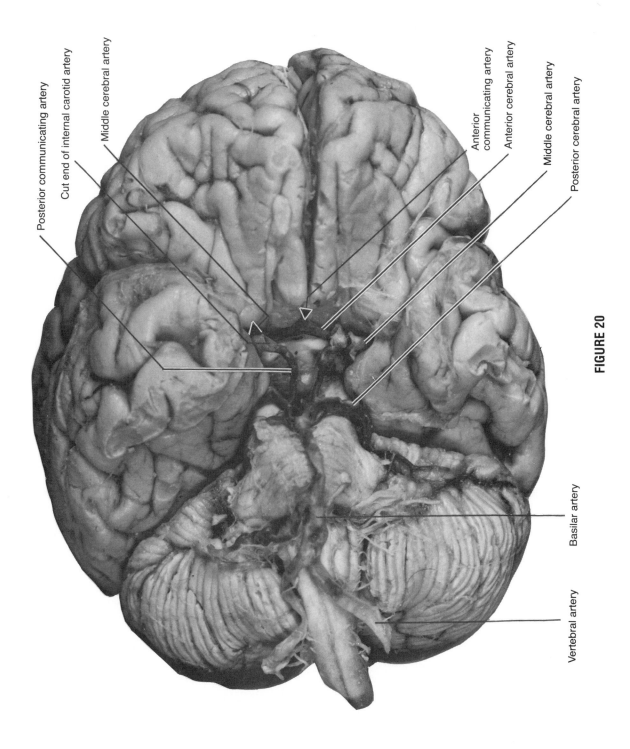

Posterior communicating artery

Cut end of internal carotid artery

Middle cerebral artery

Anterior communicating artery

Anterior cerebral artery

Middle cerebral artery

Posterior cerebral artery

Basilar artery

Vertebral artery

FIGURE 20

49

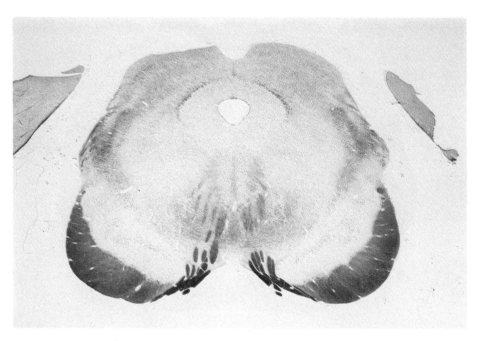

Color Figure 28. Superior colliculus cross section (B1).

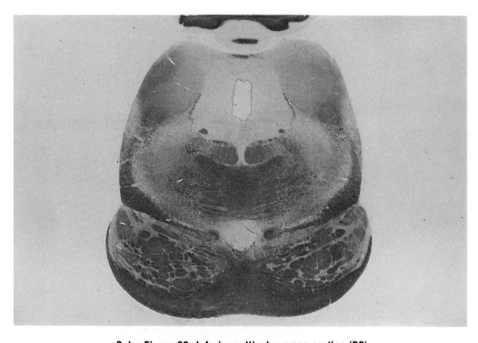

Color Figure 29. Inferior colliculus cross section (B2).

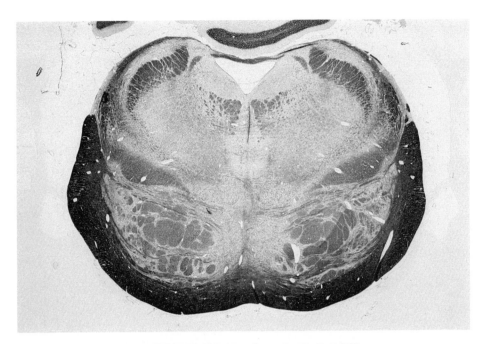

Color Figure 30. Upper pontine cross section (B3).

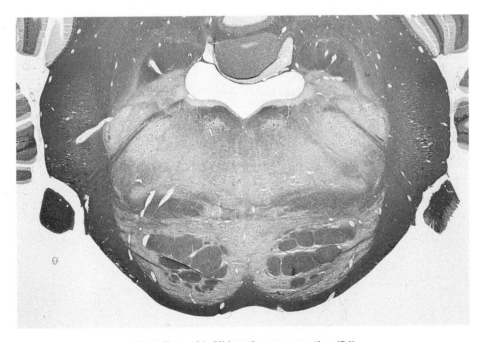

Color Figure 31. Midpontine cross section (B4).

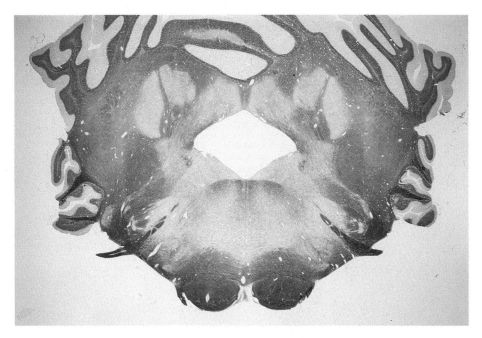

Color Figure 32. Lower pontine cross section (B5).

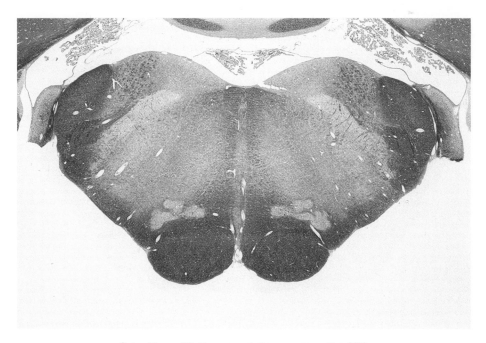

Color Figure 33. Upper medullary cross section (B6).

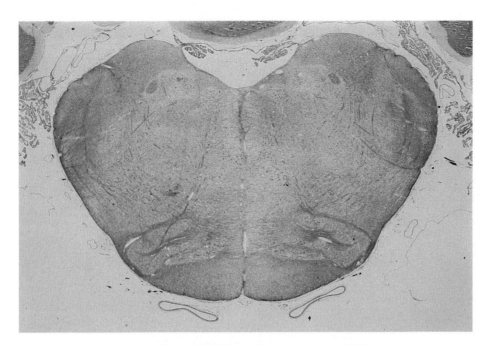

Color Figure 34. Midmedullary cross section (B7).

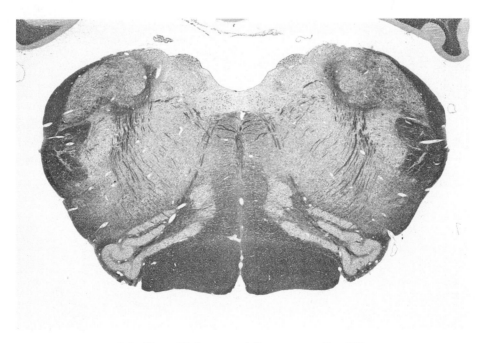

Color Figure 35. Lower medullary cross section (B8).

. . . .

Brain Stem: Cranial Nerves and Cross Sections (Figures 21–35)

INTRODUCTION

After studying the hemispheres of the brain, the next region for consideration ought to be the diencephalon. The brain stem is presented next because understanding almost all of the sensory and motor systems depends on knowledge of this part of the central nervous system (CNS). This section is followed by the sensory and motor pathways (Section C), after which the thalamic part of the diencephalon is presented (Section D). (The hypothalamus is considered with the limbic system in Section G.)

The brain stem is probably the most difficult portion of the CNS to understand. It is a relatively small mass of tissue that is packed with various nuclei and tracts. First, it is the site of origin or termination of 10 of the cranial nerves (CN III to CN XII). All the ascending pathways pass through the brain stem. Most of the motor pathways either originate in or go through it. In addition, many of the connections to the cerebellum include pathways and nuclei found in the brain stem. It is hard to imagine how all these structures actually fit into this small piece of brain tissue, which increases the difficulty of understanding this part of the brain.

Knowledge of the brain stem is necessary during the study of almost all parts of the CNS. As would be expected, this information is essential for the diagnosis of clinical syndromes that involve this part of the brain. A lesion might interrupt a sensory or motor pathway. Because of the close relationship with the cerebellum, there may be cerebellar signs as well. The accompanying cranial nerve deficits would assist a neurologist to pinpoint the brain stem level involved.

The brain stem is divided anatomically into three parts (from above downward)—the *midbrain,* the *pons,* and the *medulla.* Each of the parts is distinct when one sees a gross brain specimen or a microscopic cross section. The nuclei will be studied in this section of the *Atlas;* the tracts that pass through this region are seen in the various cross sections, and these will be studied in Section C. What makes the brain stem so difficult to understand is that these nuclei and tracts do not remain in a constant position throughout the brain stem. Not only do some of these structures change their position, but nuclei found at one level are not present at another level and are replaced by other structures. Therefore, each cross section is unique and should be studied separately. Some or all of the following structures may be present at any level:

1. Nuclei
   a. Cranial nerve nuclei of different functional types, including both sensory and motor nuclei. Knowledge of the attachment of each cranial nerve to the brain stem is a marker to the location of the cranial nerve nucleus within the brain stem in almost all cases.

    b. Nuclei connected with the cerebellum. In the midbrain, this is the red nucleus; in the pons, the pontine nuclei; in the medulla, the inferior olive. (There are others, but these three are the only ones considered here.)

    c. The reticular formation, a diffuse set of nuclei that occupy the core region of the brain stem. These are perhaps the oldest nuclei of the brain stem.

    d. Special nuclei. Those associated with sensory systems include the superior and inferior colliculi in the midbrain, nuclei involved with the auditory and vestibular systems in the medulla and pons, and the gracilis and cuneatus nuclei in the lowermost medulla. The red nucleus and the substantia nigra, both located in the midbrain, form part of the motor system.

2. Tracts

    a. Ascending tracts, to the thalamus. These include the sensory tracts related to the somatosensory and trigeminal systems, as well as the auditory pathway.

    b. Descending tracts, the largest of which is the fiber systems descending from the cortex as the corticobulbar, corticopontine, and corticospinal tracts. Other tracts that originate in the brain stem come from the red nucleus (rubrospinal); from the lateral vestibular nucleus (lateral vestibulospinal); and as two separate tracts from the reticular formation (pontine and medullary reticulospinal).

    c. Cerebellum-related tracts. Information to and from the cerebellum involves three cerebellar peduncles: the superior, attached to the midbrain; the middle, attached to the pons; and the inferior, attached to the medulla.

    d. Special tracts of the brain stem, such as the medial longitudinal fasciculus (MLF). This tract interconnects the various nuclei of the vestibular system and those associated with the eye muscles with the motor nuclei controlling the movements of the head and neck.

The ventricular system of the brain is also present throughout the brain stem (see Figs. 10A and 10B). The aqueduct goes through the midbrain and becomes the fourth ventricle; this widens and separates the pons and medulla anteriorly from the cerebellum posteriorly.

Most atlases remove the cerebellum from sections. A representative sample of the cerebellum is included with the cross sections because this may help the student to correlate these sections with the actual brain specimen, and with radiologic images of the brain, such as computed tomography (CT) scans and magnetic resonance images (MRI).

In all, the brain stem will be studied by a series of eight cross sections—two through the midbrain, three through the pons, and three through the medulla. (The actual material is based on cross sections of the monkey brain stem, which is very similar to that of the human.) The student should begin by concentrating on the names and location of the various nuclei. The tracts will be studied systematically in Section C, and the relevant cross sections will be shown again when studying the ascending and descending pathways.

Recommendation for the student: One way of facilitating the learning of material such as neuroanatomy is with color. It is suggested that the student actually color in the various nuclei and tracts by following the color guide for this section, which is found at the front of this book (see p. ix). The numbers in parentheses beside the labeled structures indicate the suggested color to be used for each of the structures. The final result will be a colored diagram, with the colors having both functional significance and consistency across sections. It is hoped that the active participation of the student in coloring the various structures will facilitate the learning of the nuclei and tracts. This act and the addition of color ought to make the material easier to understand and remember.

Color Photographs

This part of the *Atlas* is followed by a number of color photographs of the brain stem. These correspond to the levels of the cross sections. Monkey brains were fixed by perfusion and then sectioned and stained. (This material was prepared by Dr. J. Szabo [deceased] and Mrs. A. Boucher.) Myelinated fibers were stained using the Klüver-Barrera luxol-fast blue stain, which stains myelinated fibers a deep blue color. Cells have been stained with a cresyl violet counterstain, resulting in a violet-reddish color for the neuronal cell bodies (the Nissl substance is violet at higher magnification, with the cell cytoplasm taking on a reddish hue). The eight cross sections have been carefully selected to match the eight levels shown in the *Atlas* and are identified by level (e.g. superior colliculus cross section, B1). The student should refer to the appropriate figure in the *Atlas* (in the example given, this is Fig. 28) to identify the pertinent structures in these photographs.

PART B-I

CRANIAL NERVES AND NUCLEI (Figures 21–27)

FIGURE 21   **Brain Stem and Diencephalon: Ventral View**
(Photographic View)

This specimen was obtained by isolating the diencephalon and brain stem from the remainder of the brain. The dissection, using a blunt instrument, has torn through the fibers of the internal capsule (seen on the left side of the photograph).

The paired diencephalon is situated atop the brain stem. The optic chiasm is located in front of the diencephalon. Behind the optic chiasm are the mammillary bodies, nuclei of the hypothalamus (see Figs. 4 and 5).

The three parts of the brain stem can be differentiated on this ventral view:

■ The *midbrain* region has two large "pillars" anteriorly, called the *cerebral peduncles*. The fossa between the peduncles is the *interpeduncular fossa*.
■ The *pontine portion* is distinguished by its bulge anteriorly, an area composed of nuclei (the pontine nuclei).
■ The *medulla* has two distinct elevations on either side of the midline, known as the *pyramids;* these consist of axons descending to the spinal cord. Behind each is a prominent bulge, the *inferior olivary nucleus.*

The fibers projecting from the cerebral cortex can be followed through various levels of the neuraxis in this diagram. Almost all of the axons traverse the internal capsule (see Fig. 17), and most of these are found in the cerebral peduncles. Those destined for the brain stem itself (corticobulbar), and for the pons (corticopontine) terminate, leaving the corticospinal fibers within the pyramids. (All these tracts will be described in detail in Section C.) The medulla ends where the corticospinal fibers cross the midline at the pyramidal decussation. Below this is the cervical spinal cord (not labeled).

Behind the brain stem is the cerebellum, and its inferior aspect is seen on this view. Two of its lobes have been identified: the tonsils, which lie adjacent to the medulla (the clinical significance of this is discussed with Fig. 59), and the flocculus, a functionally important part of the cerebellum. The cerebellar peduncles are the connections between the brain stem and the cerebellum, and there are three pairs of them (which are described in detail with the cerebellum in Section E). In this view, two of them can be seen—the inferior cerebellar peduncle attaching the medulla and the cerebellum, and the middle cerebellar peduncle from the pons to the cerebellum.

One of the keys to understanding the brain stem is locating the cranial nerve (CN) nuclei (see Figs. 23 and 24). Unfortunately, not all of the cranial nerves have been preserved on this specimen because stripping of the meninges often tears them off (see Figs. 23–26).

■ CN III (the oculomotor nerve) emerges from the interpeduncular fossa.
■ CN IV (the trochlear nerve), which exits posteriorly, is a thin nerve that wraps around the lowermost border of the cerebral peduncle (seen on the right side in the photograph).
■ CN V (the trigeminal nerve [not labeled]) is a massive nerve attached along the middle cerebellar peduncle (see Figs. 4 and 23).
■ CN VI (the abducens nerve) is seen exiting at the junction between the pons and medulla. (It is preserved only on the left side on the photograph.)
■ CN VII (the facial nerve) has been torn; it is attached to the brain stem just above CN VIII (the acoustic nerve), at the pontocerebellar angle.
■ CN IX (the glossopharyngeal nerve), CN X (the vagus nerve), and CN XI (the spinal accessory nerve) cannot be seen on this view of the brain stem. They are attached to the lateral margin of the medulla, behind the inferior olive.
■ CN XII (the hypoglossal nerve) emerges by a series of rootlets between the inferior olive and the pyramid (preserved only on the left side in the photograph).

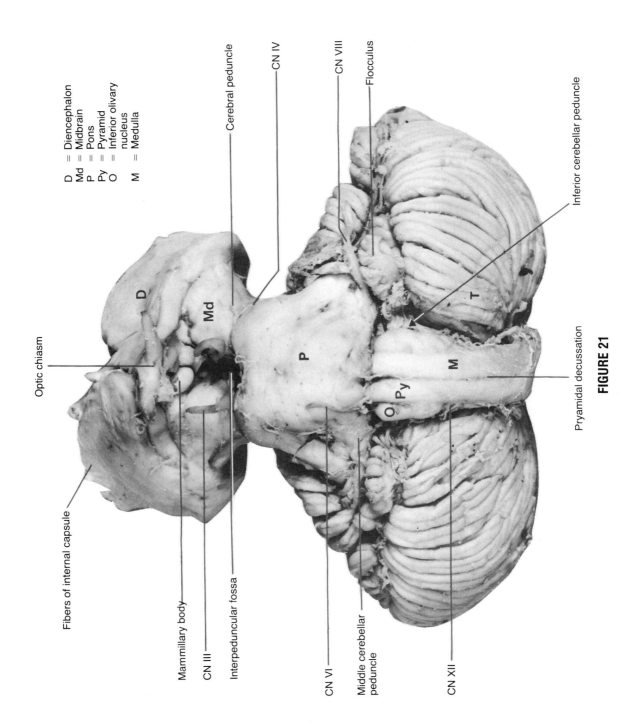

D = Diencephalon
Md = Midbrain
P = Pons
Py = Pyramid
O = Inferior olivary nucleus
M = Medulla

Optic chiasm

Cerebral peduncle

CN IV

CN VIII

Flocculus

Inferior cerebellar peduncle

Fibers of internal capsule

Mammillary body

CN III

Interpeduncular fossa

CN VI

Middle cerebellar peduncle

CN XII

Pryamidal decussation

FIGURE 21

FIGURE 22   # Brain Stem and Diencephalon: Dorsal View
(Photographic View)

This is the same specimen that was shown in Fig. 21, but it is turned around and viewed from its posterior aspect.

The diencephalon is seen as a paired structure (see Fig. 52), with one thalamus situated on either side of the third ventricle. The cut ends of the fibers of the internal capsule are again seen. Emerging from the posterior edge of the third ventricle is the pineal body.

Below the pineal are four elevations, called *colliculi,* which belong to the midbrain. The upper ones are the *superior colliculi,* and they are functionally part of the visual system. The lower (smaller) ones are the *inferior colliculi,* and these are relay nuclei in the auditory pathway. An elevation (not labeled) is seen leading away (laterally) from the inferior colliculus; this is the *brachium of the inferior colliculus,* part of the auditory pathway (see Fig. 55).

The trochlear nerve, CN IV, emerges from the brain stem dorsally, just below the inferior colliculi. These are very thin nerves and are usually lost when removing the meninges from the specimen. After emerging, they course anteriorly and follow the lowermost edge of the cerebral peduncle (see Fig. 21).

The superior aspect of the cerebellum is seen on this dorsal view. In the midline is a raised portion known as the *vermis.* One of the fissures has been opened up, the *primary fissure* anteriorly. The *horizontal fissure* is also seen at the boundary between the superior and inferior surfaces of the cerebellum. (The cerebellum will be discussed in Section E.)

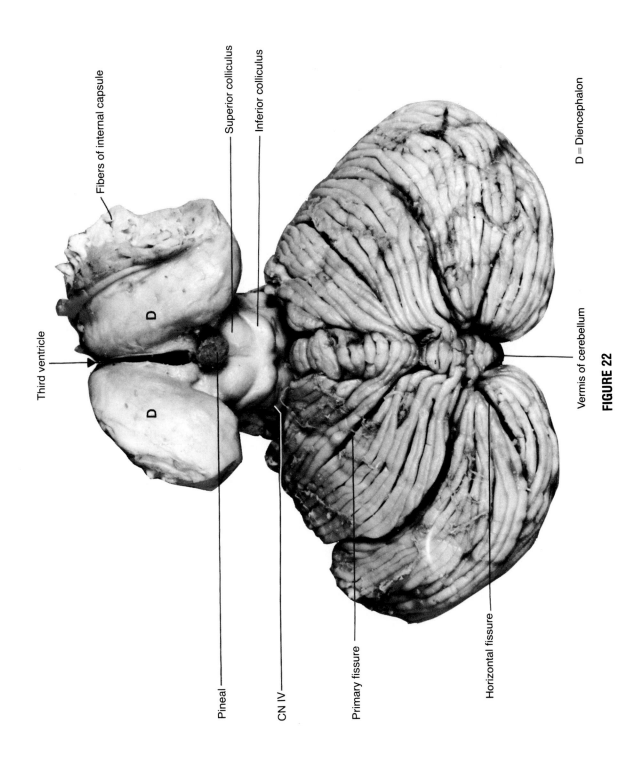

Fibers of internal capsule

Superior colliculus

Inferior colliculus

Third ventricle

D

D

Pineal

CN IV

Primary fissure

Horizontal fissure

Vermis of cerebellum

D = Diencephalon

FIGURE 22

57

FIGURE 23

Cranial Nerve Nuclei: Motor Aspects

Each of the cranial nerves may have one or more functional components—sensory, motor, or both. The motor aspects are reviewed in this diagram; the sensory ones are considered in the next diagram.

On the motor side, there are three kinds of motor functions:

- The motor supply to the muscles derived from somites (somatic motor), including nerves III, IV, VI, and XII
- The motor supply to the muscles derived from the branchial arches (branchiomotor), including nerves V, VII, IX, and X (and the cranial part of XI)
- The parasympathetic supply to smooth muscles and glands of the head and neck, including nerves III, VII, IX, and X

This diagram shows the location of the motor nuclei of the cranial nerves, superimposed on the ventral view of the brain stem. It should be apparent that only a select number of cross sections through the brain stem contain the nuclei and that different nuclei are seen at different levels. These nuclei are also shown in Fig. 48, in which the brain stem is presented from a dorsal perspective.

MIDBRAIN LEVEL

The somatic motor nucleus of the oculomotor nerve (CN III), which supplies most of the muscles of the eye, is found at the upper midbrain level. This is the level of the superior colliculus. The parasympathetic nucleus of CN III, also known as the *Edinger-Westphal nucleus,* is intermingled with a portion of the nucleus of CN III. The trochlear nucleus (CN IV), which supplies the superior oblique muscle, is found at the lower midbrain level, the level of the inferior colliculus.

PONTINE LEVEL

The motor nucleus of the trigeminal nerve (CN V) is found at the midpontine level. This branchiomotor nucleus supplies the muscles of mastication. The somatic motor nucleus of the abducens nerve (CN VI), which supplies the lateral rectus muscle, is located in the lower pontine region. Also located at this level is the bronchiomotor nucleus of CN VII, the facial nerve; this supplies the muscles of facial expression, which are derived from the branchial arches.

MEDULLARY LEVEL

CN IX and CN X are attached to the medulla along its lateral margin, behind the inferior olive. CN IX (the glossopharyngeal) and CN X (the vagus) are very complex nerves. Both have a branchiomotor component, which supplies the muscles of the pharynx (CN IX) and larynx (CN X), originating from the *nucleus ambiguus*. In addition, each has a parasympathetic component; the *dorsal motor nucleus* of the vagus innervates the organs of the thorax and abdomen. Two small parasympathetic nuclei are also shown but are rarely identified in actual brain sections. They are named the superior and inferior salivatory nuclei. The superior nucleus supplies secretomotor fibers for CN VII (to the submandibular and sublingual salivary glands, as well as nasal and lacrimal glands). The inferior nucleus supplies the same fibers for CN IX (to the parotid gland).

CN XI, the spinal accessory nerve, has two portions. The cranial part (not shown) is usually considered part of the vagus (discussed also with Fig. 48). The cervical or spinal component, which originates from a cell group in the upper four or five segments of the cervical spinal cord, supplies the large muscles of the neck (the sternomastoid and trapezius).

The somatic motor nucleus of the hypoglossal nerve (CN XII) is situated alongside the midline, throughout most of the medulla except the upper part. Its fibers exit between the pyramid and the olive, innervating all the muscles of the tongue. (**Note:** In the diagram it appears that the nucleus ambiguus is supplying the fibers to CN XII. This is merely a visualization problem; see Fig. 48.)

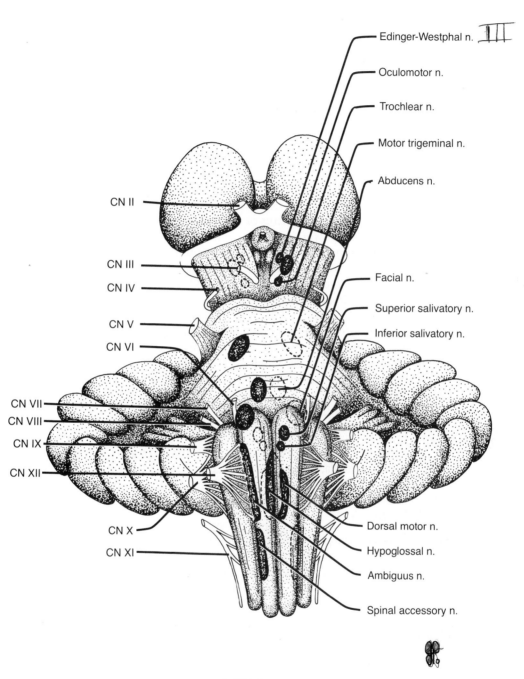

Edinger-Westphal n. |||
Oculomotor n.
Trochlear n.
Motor trigeminal n.
Abducens n.

CN II

CN III
CN IV

CN V
CN VI

Facial n.
Superior salivatory n.
Inferior salivatory n.

CN VII
CN VIII
CN IX
CN XII

CN X
CN XI

Dorsal motor n.
Hypoglossal n.
Ambiguus n.

Spinal accessory n.

FIGURE 23

FIGURE 24   # Cranial Nerve Nuclei: Sensory Aspects

Sensory information from the region of the head and neck includes the following:

- General sensations, consisting of touch (both discriminative and crude touch), pain, and temperature. These come from the skin and the mucous membranes of the mouth and the nose via branches of the trigeminal nerve.
- Sensory input from the pharynx and larynx and from the organs of the thorax and abdomen. This afferent input is carried mainly by the vagus nerve, with some coming also with the glossopharyngeal nerve. These are also called *visceral afferents*.
- Special senses, consisting of auditory and vestibular afferents, as well as the special sense of taste.

The sensory nuclei are also shown in Fig. 47, which presents the brain stem from a dorsal (posterior) perspective. It should be noted that the olfactory nerve (CN I) and the optic nerve (CN II) are not attached to the brain stem and are not considered at this stage.

TRIGEMINAL NERVE

The major sensory nerve of the head region is the trigeminal nerve (CN V) through its three divisions. The sensory components of the trigeminal nerve are found at several levels of the brain stem. The *principal (main) nucleus,* which is responsible for the discriminative aspects of touch, is located at the midpontine level, adjacent to the motor nucleus of CN V. Extending caudally from this region is a long column of cells that relay pain and temperature information from the teeth, the oral mucosa, and the skin of the face. This cell group, known as the *spinal nucleus of V,* or the *descending trigeminal nucleus,* reaches the upper cervical levels of the spinal cord (see Fig. 47).

Another group of cells extends into the midbrain region, the *mesencephalic nucleus of V*. It is an unusual cell type for the CNS in that its cells appear to be morphologically similar to neurons of the dorsal root ganglia. These neurons are thought to be the sensory proprioceptive neurons for the muscles of mastication. (The trigeminal tracts are shown in Figs. 38 and 54.)

VISCERAL AFFERENTS AND TASTE

The nucleus that receives the visceral afferents from CN IX and CN X is the *solitary nucleus*. It is found in the medulla, medial to the spinal trigeminal nucleus. The special sense of taste, mainly carried in CN VII, as well as in CN IX and CN X, also synapses in the solitary nucleus.

COCHLEAR NUCLEI

The auditory fibers from the spiral ganglion are carried to the CNS in CN VIII, then branch and form their first synapses in the *dorsal* and *ventral cochlear nuclei* (depicted diagrammatically as one nucleus). These nuclei are situated along the course of the nerve as it enters the brain stem (see Fig. 47). Tonotopic localization is maintained in these nuclei. (The auditory pathway is shown in Figs. 39 and 55.)

VESTIBULAR NUCLEI

Vestibular afferents enter the CNS as part of CN VIII. The vestibular nuclei are located in the upper medullary level as well as the lower pontine level. There are four nuclei—the *medial* and *inferior* nuclei located in the medulla, the *lateral* nucleus located at the pontomedullary junction, and the small *superior* nucleus located in the lower pontine region (shown also in Fig. 51). The vestibular afferents terminate in these nuclei. The lateral vestibular nucleus, which has giant neurons, is the origin of the lateral vestibulospinal tract (see Fig. 43). Some of the fibers of the medial longitudinal fasciculus (MLF) are derived from the other vestibular nuclei (discussed with Fig. 51).

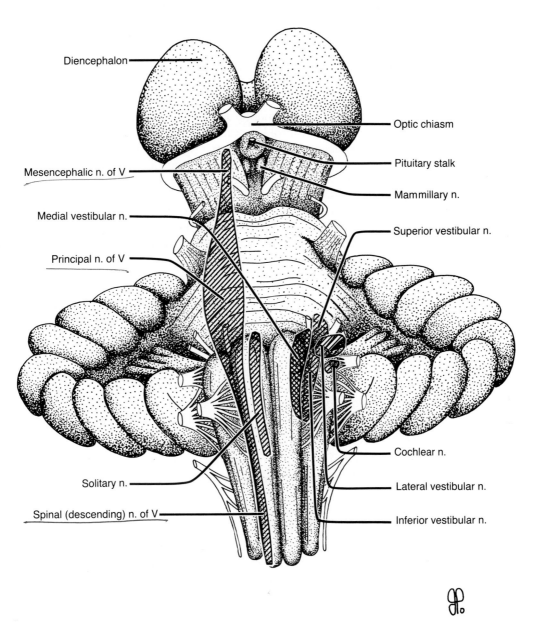

Diencephalon

Optic chiasm

Pituitary stalk

Mesencephalic n. of V

Mammillary n.

Medial vestibular n.

Superior vestibular n.

Principal n. of V

Cochlear n.

Solitary n.

Lateral vestibular n.

Spinal (descending) n. of V

Inferior vestibular n.

FIGURE 24

61

FIGURE 25 # Reticular Formation

The reticular formation is the name for a group of neurons found throughout the brain stem. It is an old set of neurons that function in a network manner. The reticular formation occupies the central portion or core area of the brain stem, from midbrain to medulla (Figs. 28 to 35).

These nuclei receive afferents from almost all the sensory systems and project to virtually all parts of the nervous system. Anatomically, there is a high degree of interconnection among the nuclei of the reticular formation. Functionally, it is possible to localize different subgroups within the reticular formation:

■ *Cardiac and respiratory centers:* Subsets of neurons within the pontine and medullary reticular formation are responsible for the control of the vital functions of heart rate and respiration.
■ *Motor functions:* Both the pontine and medullary nuclei of the reticular formation contribute to motor control by means of the corticoreticulospinal system (Figs. 44 and 45). In addition, these nuclei exert a significant influence on muscle tone.
■ *Ascending projection system:* Fibers from the reticular formation ascend to the thalamus and project to various nonspecific thalamic nuclei. From these nuclei, fibers are distributed diffusely to the cerebral cortex. This whole system is concerned with consciousness and has been called the *ascending reticular activating system.*
■ *Precerebellar nuclei:* Numerous nuclei in the brain stem are located within the boundaries of the reticular formation and project to the cerebellum. These are not always included in discussions of the reticular formation.

The nuclei of the reticular formation are also shown in Fig. 49, a view of the brain stem from the dorsal perspective.

It is also possible to describe the reticular formation topographically. The neurons appear to be arranged in three longitudinal sets (these are shown in the lefthand side of the figure):

■ The lateral group consists of small neurons. These are thought to be the neurons that receive the various inputs to the reticular formation.
■ The next group of neurons (medially) is called the central group. These cells are larger and project their axons upward and downward. Within this group are the well-known *nucleus gigantocellularis* of the medulla and the *nuclei pontis,* caudal and oral portions, located in the lower and upper pontine levels.
■ A set of neurons occupies the midline region of the brain stem; these neurons are called the *raphe nuclei.* The best-known nucleus of this group is the *nucleus raphe magnus,* which plays an important role in the descending pain system (see Fig. 50).

In addition, both the *locus ceruleus* and the *periaqueductal gray* are considered part of the reticular formation (discussed with Fig. 49).

In summary, the reticular formation is a phylogenetically old system that is connected with almost all parts of the CNS. Although it has a generalized influence within the CNS, it also contains subsystems that are directly involved in specific CNS functions.

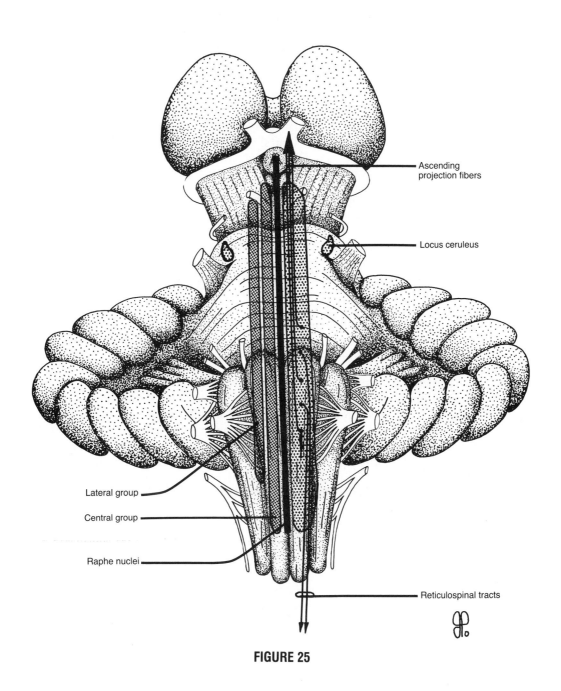

Ascending
projection fibers

Locus ceruleus

Lateral group

Central group

Raphe nuclei

Reticulospinal tracts

FIGURE 25

FIGURE 26

Ventral View of the Brain Stem

This diagram is similar to the photographic view of the brain stem (see Fig. 21).

Study of the brain stem will be continued by examining its histologic anatomy through a series of cross sections. Since it is well beyond the scope of the nonspecialist to know all the details, certain salient points have been selected, including the cranial nerve nuclei, the ascending and descending tracts, certain brain stem nuclei that belong to the reticular formation, and other special nuclei.

As has been indicated, the attachment of the cranial nerves to the brain stem is one of the keys to being able to understand this part of the brain. Wherever a cranial nerve is attached to the brain stem, its nucleus (or some of its nuclei) is located at that level. Therefore, if one memorizes the attachment of the cranial nerves to the brain stem, one has a key to its understanding.

Since the focus is on the cranial nerves, only a limited number of cross sections will be studied. This diagram shows the ventral view of the brain stem, with the attached cranial nerves, and indicates the sections depicted in the series to follow. There are eight cross sections taken at the following levels:

- Two through the midbrain:
    B1—CN III, superior colliculus level
    B2—CN IV, inferior colliculus level
- Three through the pons:
    B3—uppermost pons (there is no cranial nerve attachment at this level)
    B4—midpons, CN V (through the principal nucleus)
    B5—CN VI, CN VII, and part of CN VIII, the lowermost pons
- Three through the medulla:
    B6—CN VIII, the uppermost medulla
    B7—CN IX, CN X, and CN XII, the midmedullary level
    B8—lowermost medulla, with some special nuclei

The letter B refers both to brain stem and to this section of the *Atlas*. Reference to these cross sections uses either the figure number or the cross-sectional level.

The information presented in this series should be sufficient to allow a student to recognize the clinical signs that would accompany a lesion at a particular level, especially as they pertain to the cranial nerves. Later on, the various pathways will be studied and this will add significant information, since almost all brain stem lesions interrupt either ascending or descending tracts. In the next section, when the tracts are being studied, reference will be made to these cross-sectional levels.

B1 ——————————————————————————

B2 ——————————————————————————

B3 ——————————————————————————

B4 ——————————————————————————

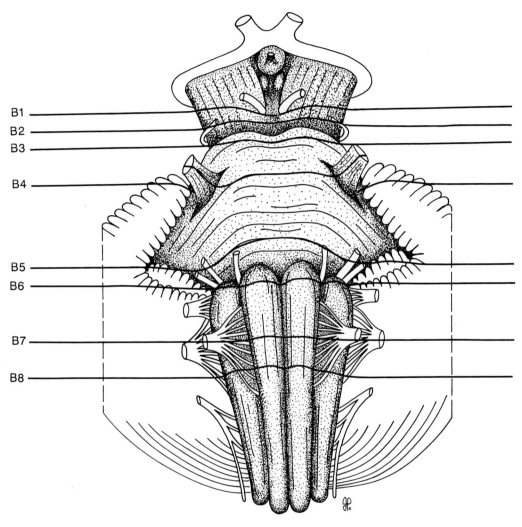

B5 ——————————————————————————

B6 ——————————————————————————

B7 ——————————————————————————

B8 ——————————————————————————

FIGURE 26

FIGURE 27   # Sagittal View of the Brain Stem

This is a schematic drawing of the brain stem seen in a midsagittal view (see Fig. 7 for a photograph of the brain in midsagittal view). This representation will be shown in each of the cross-sectional diagrams, with the exact level indicated, to orient the student to the level of the cross section.

This view is being presented because it is commonly used to portray the brain stem. It should be correlated with the ventral view shown in the previous diagram. The location of some nuclei of the brain stem can be easily visualized using this sagittal view, including the red nucleus in the midbrain, the pontine nuclei that form the bulging "potbelly" of the pons, and the inferior olivary nucleus of the medulla.

Using this orientation, one can approach the description of the eight cross sections systematically:

- The most anterior portion of each part of the brain stem contains some representation of the descending cortical fibers, specifically the corticobulbar, corticopontine, and corticospinal pathways (see Figs. 40 and 48). In the midbrain, the cerebral peduncles include all these axon systems. The corticobulbar fibers are given off to the various brain stem and cranial nerve nuclei. (*Bulb* is the alternate term for the brain stem.) In the pons, the corticopontine fibers terminate in the pontine nuclei, which form the bulge known as the *pons proper*. In the medulla, the corticospinal fibers form the *pyramids*. The medulla ends at the point where these fibers decussate (see Fig. 21).
- The central portion of the brain stem is called the *tegmentum*. The reticular formation occupies the core region of the tegmentum. This area contains the cranial nerve nuclei, as well as other nuclei, including the red nucleus and the inferior olive, and all the remaining tracts.
- The ventricular system has been indicated with stippling. Therefore, the sections can be oriented according to the parts of the ventricular system that pass through this region—the aqueduct in the midbrain region and the fourth ventricle farther down (see Figs. 10A and 10B).
- It is evident that the colliculi are located behind the aqueduct of the midbrain, and that the fourth ventricle separates the pons and medulla from the cerebellum. The upper part of the roof of the fourth ventricle is called the *superior medullary velum* (see Figs. 7 and 46). The location of the choroid plexus in the inferior aspect of the roof of the fourth ventricle is also shown.

Note: The brain stem is being described starting from the midbrain through to the medulla for two reasons:

1 This order follows the numbering of the cranial nerves, from above downward.
2 This is the sequence that has been described for the fibers descending from the cortex.

Others may prefer to start the description of the cross sections from the medulla upward.

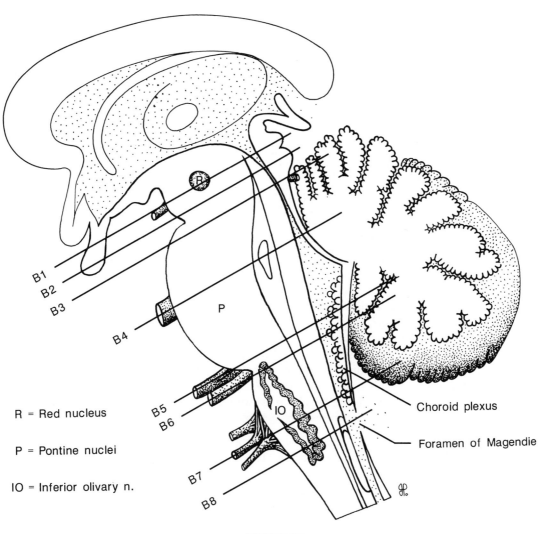

B1
B2
B3
B4
B5
B6
B7
B8

R = Red nucleus

P = Pontine nuclei

IO = Inferior olivary n.

P

IO

Choroid plexus

Foramen of Magendie

FIGURE 27

PART B-II

THE MIDBRAIN (Figures 28 and 29)

The midbrain is the smallest of the three parts of the brain stem. Often, it is not really seen on an inferior view of the brain because the temporal lobes of the hemispheres tend to obscure it (see Fig. 4).

The midbrain area is easily recognizable from the anterior view in a dissected specimen (see Fig. 21). Most anteriorly are the massive *cerebral peduncles*. The peduncles contain axons that are a direct continuation of the fiber systems of the internal capsule (see Fig. 17). Within them are the pathways descending from the cerebral cortex to the brain stem, the cerebellum via the pons, and the spinal cord—the corticobulbar, corticopontine, and corticospinal tracts (see Figs. 40 and 48).

In a midsagittal section of the brain and brain stem (see Figs. 7 and 27), the midbrain area is easily identified as the part containing the cerebral aqueduct. Posterior to the aqueduct are the two pair of colliculi, which can also be seen on the dorsal view of the isolated brain stem (see Fig. 22). The four nuclei together form the *tectal plate*, or *tectum*. The *superior colliculus* is a subcortical center for certain visual reflexes. These nuclei give rise to a fiber tract, the *tectospinal tract*, that descends to the cervical spinal cord as part of the medial longitudinal fasciculus (discussed with Fig. 51). The system is involved in the coordination of the movements of the eyes with those of the head and neck, both of these responding to visual and vestibular afferents. The *inferior colliculus* is a relay nucleus in the auditory pathway and is discussed with this system (see Figs. 39 and 55).

There are two distinct nuclei in the midbrain region—the substantia nigra and the red nucleus.

■ The *substantia nigra* is found throughout the midbrain and is located behind the cerebral peduncles (see Fig. 15). It derives its name from the dark, melaninlike pigment found within its neurons in freshly dissected specimens of human material (see Fig. 5; the nucleus has thus been color coded in black). This is an important nucleus in the regulation of movements. The substantia nigra is functionally part of the basal ganglia, with which it has interconnections. Some of its neurons produce dopamine, a distinct neurotransmitter. Loss of these neurons results in the clinical entity Parkinson's disease (discussed with Fig. 12). It is important to realize that, despite its name, this nuclear area is clear (white) in most photographs in atlases. This is because the pigment is not retained when the specimen is processed: with myelin-type stains, the area appears empty; with cell stains, the neurons are visible.

■ The *red nucleus* is located in the *tegmentum,* the inner region of the brain stem. The label *red* is derived from the fact that this nucleus is sometimes reddish in a freshly dissected specimen, presumably because of its marked vascularity. (This nucleus has thus been color coded in red.) The red nucleus is found at the level of the superior colliculus. It gives rise to a fiber tract that descends to the spinal cord, the *rubrospinal tract* (see Fig. 42).

The substantia nigra, the red nucleus, and the superior colliculus are all involved with more integrative aspects of motor control.

The *pretectal region* is located in front and somewhat above the superior colliculus. This region is the center for the reflex response of the pupil to light, the *pupillary light reflex.* The reflex requires input from receptors in the retina, and the output occurs through the parasympathetic neurons in the Edinger-Westphal nucleus (see Fig. 23) and the oculomotor nerve (CN III). Light shone on one eye normally leads to a rapid constriction of the pupil on the same side and a similar reaction on the other side, the *consensual response.* The coordination of the responses of the two sides is by means of commissural fibers (in the posterior commissure; see Fig. 51). Because the pupillary light reflex is one of the most important reflexes to test clinically, particularly in head-injured and comatose patients, knowledge of this pathway and the areas involved is essential.

The reticular formation is found in the core area of the tegmentum. The reticular formation of the midbrain is particularly important for the maintenance of consciousness. A rather special part of the reticular formation at this level is the periaqueductal gray that surrounds the aqueduct. This region forms part of the descending control system for pain modulation (see Fig. 50).

Some lesions may destroy much of the brain stem yet leave the midbrain intact (e.g., a thrombosis of the basilar artery). This may allow the patient to survive in a particular (rather tragic) state. Usually, all voluntary movements are gone, except for some eye movements. Likewise, there is a loss of sensation. The patient is left in a state of consciousness with intellectual functions generally intact. The whole clinical picture is known by the name *locked-in syndrome.*

Two levels are needed for a study of the brain stem:

■ The upper (*rostral*) one passes through the nucleus of CN III and the superior colliculus.
■ The lower (*caudal*) one is at the level of the nucleus of CN IV and the inferior colliculus.

FIGURE 28

Superior Colliculus Cross Section (B1)

In a cross section of the brain stem through the rostral midbrain, the most ventral (anterior) structure is the cerebral peduncle. Posterior to it is the substantia nigra. The superior colliculus is located dorsally, behind the aqueduct. The region surrounding the aqueduct of the midbrain (the aqueduct of Sylvius) is the periaqueductal gray.

Within the cerebral peduncles, the fiber systems are segregated: the corticobulbar and particularly the corticospinal pathways occupy its middle third, while the outer and inner portions carry the corticopontine fibers (see Figs. 40 and 48).

The substantia nigra is seen to have two parts that are functionally distinct—the pars compacta and pars reticulata. The *pars reticulata* lies adjacent to the cerebral peduncle and contains some widely dispersed neurons. Located more dorsally, the *pars compacta* is a cell-rich region whose neurons contain the melaninlike pigment (see Fig. 5); these are the dopaminergic neurons that project to the neostriatum (see Fig. 15).

The *oculomotor nucleus* is large and occupies the region in front of the periaqueductal gray, near the midline; this is the typical location for all nuclei that are efferent to somatic muscles. These motor neurons are large and easily recognizable. The parasympathetic portion of this nucleus is incorporated within it and is known as the *Edinger-Westphal nucleus* (see Fig. 23). The fibers of CN III exit anteriorly between the cerebral peduncles, in the *interpeduncular fossa*.

The *red nucleus* is located within the tegmentum. With a section that has been stained for myelin, it is seen as a clear zone. With a cell-type stain, one can discern the outline of the nucleus. The fibers of CN III exit through the medial portion of this nucleus. The red nucleus gives origin to a descending pathway, the *rubrospinal tract* (Figs. 42 and 48), which is involved in motor control. This pathway is not thought to play as important a role in the overall functioning of the motor system in humans compared with other mammals and higher apes.

The *superior colliculus* gives rise to a descending pathway (the tectospinal tract) that is involved in the control of eye and neck movements. Functionally, these fibers can be considered part of the *medial longitudinal fasciculus* (MLF; see Fig. 51). In fact, this descending pathway travels with the MLF throughout the brain stem and upper spinal cord. The MLF stains heavily with a myelin-type stain and is found anterior to the somatic motor nucleus, next to the midline, at this level and at the other levels of the brain stem.

The ascending tracts present in the midbrain are a continuation of those present throughout the brain stem. The medial lemniscus, the ascending trigeminal pathways, and the fibers of the anterolateral system incorporated with them are on their way to the thalamus (see Figs. 47 and 54).

Also visible at this level is the brachium of the inferior colliculus, a part of the auditory pathway. This fiber bundle connects the inferior colliculus to the medial geniculate nucleus of the thalamus. It is situated close to the surface on the dorsal aspect (see Figs. 22 and 55).

Note: The suggested colors for coding the various nuclei and tracts are indicated in parentheses beside the labeled structures. Please refer to the front of this book (p. ix) for the color coding.

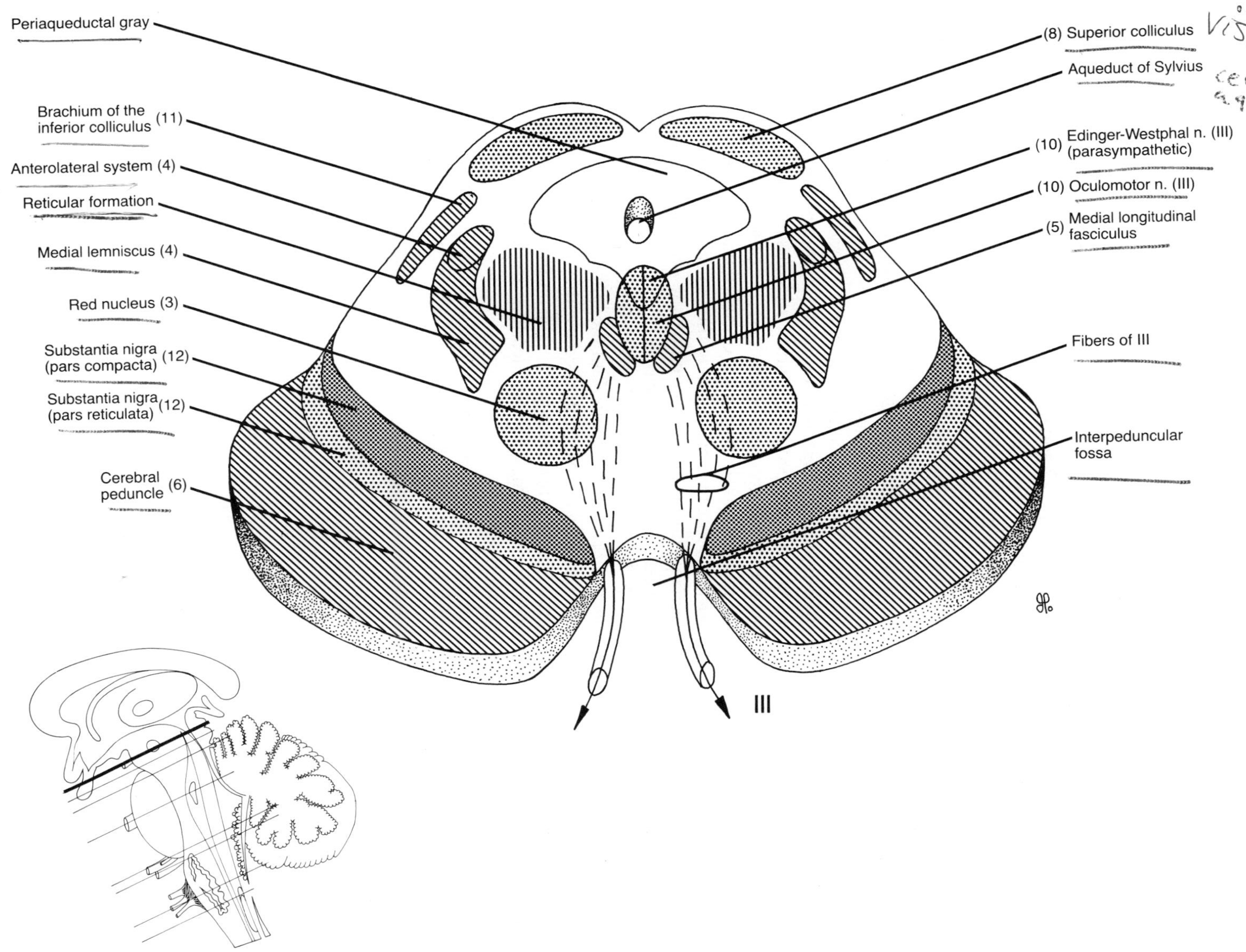

Periaqueductal gray

Brachium of the
inferior colliculus (11)

Anterolateral system (4)

Reticular formation

Medial lemniscus (4)

Red nucleus (3)

Substantia nigra
(pars compacta) (12)

Substantia nigra
(pars reticulata) (12)

Cerebral
peduncle (6)

(8) Superior colliculus

Aqueduct of Sylvius

(10) Edinger-Westphal n. (III)
(parasympathetic)

(10) Oculomotor n. (III)

(5) Medial longitudinal
fasciculus

Fibers of III

Interpeduncular
fossa

III

Visual
cerebral
aqueduct

(pain)

(pain)

FIGURE 28

71

FIGURE 29   # Inferior Colliculus Cross Section (B2)

This is a cross section of the brain stem through the caudal midbrain. The cerebral peduncles are still located anteriorly. The substantia nigra is located immediately behind these fibers. Dorsal to the cerebral aqueduct is the inferior colliculus.

The inferior colliculus is a relay nucleus in the auditory pathway. The ascending auditory fibers, collectively called the *lateral lemniscus,* are still present at this level and are often seen terminating in this nucleus (see Figs. 39 and 55).

The nucleus of CN IV, the *trochlear nucleus,* is located in front of the periaqueductal gray, next to the midline. Because it supplies only one extraocular muscle, it is a smaller nucleus than the oculomotor nucleus. CN IV proceeds dorsally and exits from the brain stem below the inferior colliculus (see Figs. 22 and 46). Its fibers cross before exiting. The MLF lies just anterior to the trochlear nucleus.

The medial lemniscus, the trigeminal fibers, and the anterolateral fibers (system) are situated at the lateral edge of the tegmentum (see Fig. 54). In fact, they are found at this level at the surface of the midbrain. In select instances, particularly with cancer patients who are suffering from intractable pain, it is possible to surgically sever the sensory ascending pathways at this level. Obviously, this rather dangerous and difficult neurosurgical procedure would be considered only as a measure of last resort.

In cross sections through the lower aspects of this region, a massive fiber system (as seen with a myelin-type stain) occupies the central region of the midbrain. These fibers are the continuation of the superior cerebellar peduncles, which are crossing (decussating) at this level. The fibers are coming from the deep cerebellar nuclei (i.e., the intracerebellar nuclei) and are headed for the red nucleus and the thalamus (discussed with Figs. 47 and 63).

The nuclei of the reticular formation are found in the central region of the brain stem (the tegmentum). The periaqueductal gray surrounding the cerebral aqueduct often has some unusually large round cells at its edges; these cells are part of the *mesencephalic nucleus* of the trigeminal nerve (CN V) (see Fig. 24). Between the cerebral peduncles is a small nucleus, the *interpeduncular nucleus,* that belongs with the limbic system.

Some cross sections at this level are confusing because they may contain some pontine nuclei. This is possible if the section is not cut exactly in the proper plane. In some cases, the pontine nuclei reach more cranially (higher) and therefore are found at the level of the lowermost portion of the midbrain.

Note: The suggested colors for coding the various nuclei and tracts are indicated in parentheses beside the labeled structures. Please refer to the front of this book (p. ix) for the color coding.

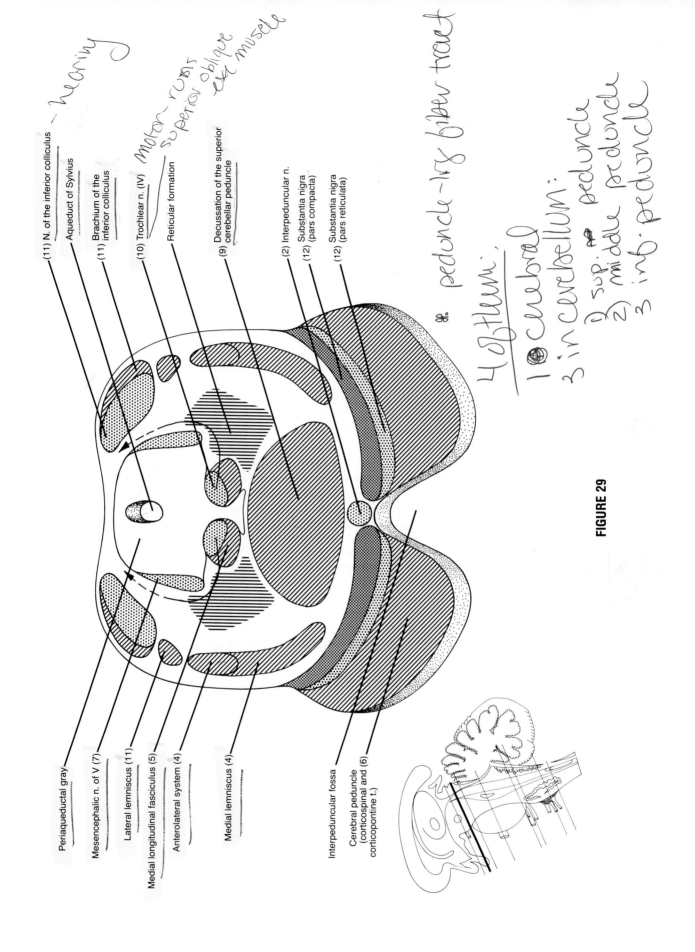

FIGURE 29

Periaqueductal gray

Mesencephalic n. of V (7)

Lateral lemniscus (11)

Medial longitudinal fasciculus (5)

Anterolateral system (4)

Medial lemniscus (4)

Interpeduncular fossa

Cerebral peduncle
(corticospinal and (6)
corticopontine t.)

(11) N. of the inferior colliculus — hearing

Aqueduct of Sylvius

(11) Brachium of the
inferior colliculus

(10) Trochlear n. (IV) — motor - runs superior oblique ext muscle

Reticular formation

(9) Decussation of the superior
cerebellar peduncle

(2) Interpeduncular n.

(12) Substantia nigra
(pars compacta)

(12) Substantia nigra
(pars reticulata)

peduncle-lrg fiber tract

4 Of Hem:
① cerebral
3 in cerebellum:
② sup. peduncle
③ middle peduncle
③ inf. peduncle

73

PART B-III

THE PONS (Figures 30–32)

The pons, medulla, and cerebellum are part of the so-called hindbrain. These structures are located in the posterior cranial fossa of the skull, along with the fourth ventricle. This ventricle separates the pons and medulla anteriorly from the cerebellum posteriorly (see Figs. 7 and 27).

The pons is characterized by its protruding anterior portion, the *pons proper*. This consists of a large group of nuclei, the *pontine nuclei*. The corticopontine fibers that descend through the cerebral peduncles terminate in these nuclei. From here, they are relayed on to the cerebellum (see Figs. 40 and 48) by means of the *middle cerebellar peduncle*. The pons proper forms a bridgelike structure between these two prominent cerebellar peduncles.

Also found intermingled with the pontine nuclei are the fiber bundles that belong to the corticospinal system. These continue through this region (without synapsing) and emerge at the medullary level to form the pyramids (see Figs. 21 and 41).

Behind the pons proper is the *tegmentum*, the region of the brain stem that contains the cranial nerve nuclei, the ascending and descending tracts, and the nuclei of the reticular formation. The cranial nerves attached to the pons include the trigeminal (CN V), the abducens (CN VI), the facial (CN VII), and part of the vestibulocochlear (CN VIII).

CN V: A review of the nuclei of the trigeminal nerve (Figs. 23, 24, and 47) indicates that parts of its nuclei are found at all levels of the pons. The midpontine section is taken at the level of the attachment of CN V, and both the principal sensory nucleus and the motor nucleus are found at this cross-sectional level.

CN VI: The abducens nerve is a typical somatic motor nucleus, innervating the lateral rectus muscle of the eye. The nucleus is located in the lowermost pons, and its fibers exit anteriorly and at a slightly lower level, at the junction of the pons and medulla (see Figs. 21 and 23).

CN VII: The facial nerve has a most unusual course within the brain stem. The fibers of CN VII form an internal loop over the abducens nucleus (see Fig. 48), ascending, looping, and then descending to exit laterally at the junction of the pons and the cerebellum, the *cerebellopontine angle*.

CN VIII: The fibers of the cochlear and vestibular divisions of CN VIII enter the brain stem adjacent to CN VII, at the cerebellopontine angle.

■ *Cochlear portion:* The auditory fibers synapse in the dorsal and ventral cochlear nuclei, which will be seen in the upper medulla cross section (see Figs. 33 and 47). After this, there is a synapse in the nuclear group called the *superior olivary complex,* which is found in the lowermost pons. Some of the fibers cross the midline before synapsing, and some cross after synapsing. The crossing fibers form a structure that is known as the *trapezoid body*. After one or more synapses, the fibers ascend and, in so doing, form a new tract, the *lateral lemniscus,* which actually commences at this level. (The auditory pathway is discussed with Figs. 39 and 55.)

- *Vestibular portion:* The vestibular nuclei are found in the lowermost pontine region and at the upper levels of the medulla (see Fig. 24). The lateral vestibular nucleus gives rise to the *lateral vestibulospinal tract* (see Fig. 43). The medial and superior vestibular nuclei contribute fibers to the MLF, relating the vestibular sensory information to eye movements (discussed with Fig. 51).

A not uncommon tumor, called an *acoustic neuroma,* can occur along the course of the acoustic nerve, usually at the cerebellopontine angle. This is a slow-growing, benign tumor composed of Schwann cells, the cell responsible for myelin in the peripheral nervous system. Initially, a person may complain of loss of hearing and perhaps a ringing noise in the ear (called *tinnitus*). Because of its location, as the tumor grows it begins to compress the adjacent nerves (including CN VII). Eventually, if the tumor is left unattended, additional symptoms occur because of further compression of the brain stem. Detection of acoustic neuromas has been made much easier using modern imaging techniques. Surgical removal, however, still requires considerable skill so as not to damage adjacent structures.

The ascending tracts present in the tegmentum convey sensory information from the body. These include the medial lemniscus and the anterolateral fibers (system). The medial lemniscus shifts its position in its course through the brain stem (see Figs. 36 and 47), moving from a central to a lateral position. The anterolateral system is too small to be identified and eventually becomes incorporated with the more easily recognized medial lemniscus (see Fig. 47).

The fourth ventricle begins in the pontine region. It starts as a widening of the aqueduct and then continues to enlarge so that it is widest at about the level of the junction between the pons and medulla. There is no pontine nucleus dorsal to the fourth ventricle. The cerebellum is located above (posterior to) the roof of the ventricle. It is at the level of the mid and lower pontine cross sections that one finds the deep cerebellar nuclei (presented in Figs. 60 and 62).

The pons is to be represented by three sections:

- *Uppermost pons:* This has been taken at the exit point of the trochlear nerve (CN IV). There are also several features here that are important in making the transition between the pons and the midbrain.
- *Middle pons:* This is at the level of the attachment of the trigeminal nerve. It includes the massive middle cerebellar peduncles.
- *Lowermost pons:* This cross section is taken just above the junction with the medulla. This lowermost level is one of the most complex cross sections of the brain stem, since it has the nuclei of CN VI, CN VII, and parts of both divisions of CN VIII.

FIGURE 30 # Upper Pontine Cross Section (B3)

This cross section of the brain stem through the rostral pons is presented mainly to allow an understanding of the transition of midbrain to pons. This particular section is taken at the uppermost pontine level, where the trochlear nerve exits (below the inferior colliculus; see Fig. 22). This is the only cranial nerve that exits posteriorly. Its fibers cross before exiting.

Anteriorly, the pontine nuclei are beginning to appear. Corticopontine fibers are terminating in the pontine nuclei. From these cells, a new tract is formed that projects to the cerebellum, the *middle cerebellar peduncle*. The corticospinal fibers are coursing in bundles between these nuclei (without synapsing).

Centrally, the cerebral aqueduct is beginning to enlarge, becoming, by definition, the *fourth ventricle*. In this section, the area is still surrounded by the periaqueductal gray. The MLF is found in its typical location ventral to the fourth ventricle, next to the midline. Nuclei of the reticular formation are present as they are throughout the brain stem.

The ascending tracts include the lateral lemniscus (auditory), the medial lemniscus and anterolateral system (somatosensory from the body), and the ascending trigeminal fibers (from the face). The auditory fibers are located dorsally, just before terminating in the inferior colliculus (in the lower midbrain, which is just superior to this level). The medial lemniscus, with the adjoining fibers of the anterolateral system, is located midway between its more central position inferiorly and the lateral position found in the midbrain (see Figs. 36 and 47). In sections stained for myelin, it has a typical comma-shaped configuration. Some of the ascending trigeminal fibers are associated with the medial lemniscus and others are not (see Fig. 54).

There is a rather special nucleus located at this level, the *locus ceruleus*. The nucleus derives its name from its bluish color in fresh specimens. (It has therefore been color coded in blue.) It is considered part of the reticular formation (as discussed with Fig. 25). This nucleus is unique because of its widespread connections with virtually all parts of the brain, and because it has noradrenaline as its neurotransmitter substance (see Fig. 49). The nucleus is located in the dorsal part of the tegmentum not too far from the edges of the fourth ventricle. Nearby may be seen some of the large neurons that belong to the *mesencephalic nucleus* of the trigeminal (see Fig. 24). Neither of these cell groups is particularly large and, unfortunately, may not be found in every cross section of this region.

The *superior cerebellar peduncle* is found within the tegmentum of the pons. These fibers carry information from the cerebellum to the red nucleus and the thalamus. The fibers, which are the axons from the deep cerebellar nuclei, leave the cerebellum and course in the roof of the fourth ventricle. They then enter the pontine region and move toward the midline, finally decussating in the lower midbrain (see Figs. 46, 47, and 63).

The uppermost part of the cerebellum is found at this level. One of the parts of the vermis, the midline portion of the cerebellum, is identified—the *lingula*. This lobule is a useful landmark in the study of the cerebellum and will be identified again when the anatomy of the cerebellum is being explained (see Fig. 58).

Note: The suggested colors for coding the various nuclei and tracts are indicated in parentheses beside the labeled structures. Please refer to the front of this book (p. ix) for the color coding.

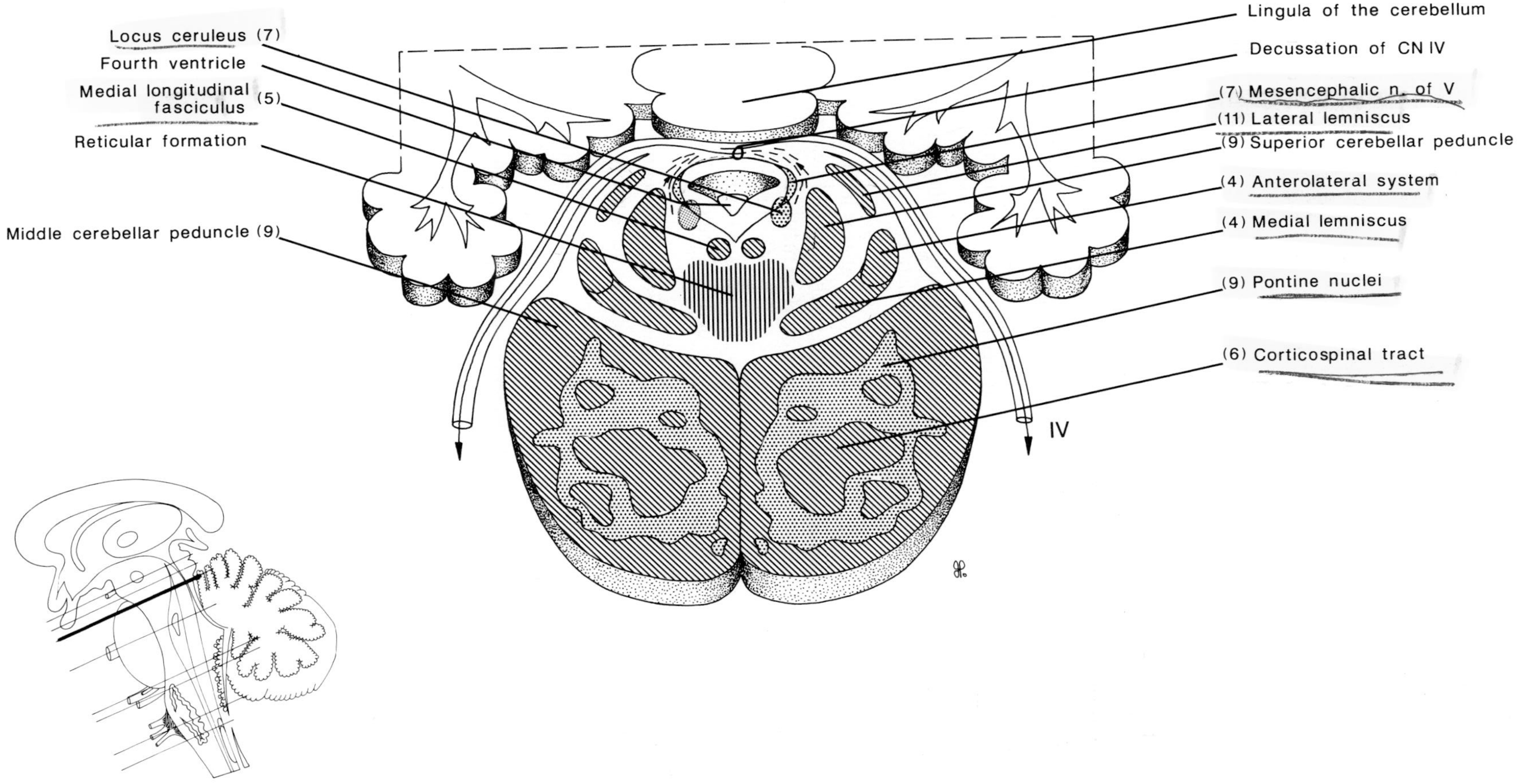

Lingula of the cerebellum

Decussation of CN IV

(7) Mesencephalic n. of V

(11) Lateral lemniscus

(9) Superior cerebellar peduncle

(4) Anterolateral system

(4) Medial lemniscus

(9) Pontine nuclei

(6) Corticospinal tract

IV

Locus ceruleus (7)

Fourth ventricle

Medial longitudinal
fasciculus (5)

Reticular formation

Middle cerebellar peduncle (9)

FIGURE 30

77

FIGURE 31

Midpontine Cross Section (B4)

This cross section of the brain stem is taken through the level of the attachment of the trigeminal nerve (CN V). Anteriorly, the pontine nuclei and the bundles of corticospinal fibers are easily recognized. The pontine cells, whose axons give rise to the middle cerebellar peduncle, are particularly numerous at this level.

The trigeminal nerve is attached along the course of the middle cerebellar peduncle. CN V has several nuclei with different functions (see Figs. 23 and 24). This level contains only two of its four nuclei—the principal (or main) sensory nucleus and the motor nucleus. The *principal (main) sensory nucleus* subserves discriminative (e.g., two-point) touch sensation and accounts for most of the fibers. The *motor nucleus* supplies the muscles of mastication and sometimes these fibers exit as a separate nerve. These nuclei are separated by the fibers of CN V; the sensory nucleus (with smaller cells) is found more laterally, and the motor nucleus (with larger cells) more medially.

The ascending fiber systems are easily located at this cross-sectional level. The medial lemniscus moves away from the midline as it ascends. The anterolateral fiber system becomes associated with it by this level (see Fig. 47). The lateral lemniscus is seen as a distinct tract situated just lateral to the medial lemniscus. The MLF is found in its typical location anterior to the ventricle.

The core area of the tegmentum is occupied by the nuclei of the reticular formation. Some of the nuclei here are called the *oral portion* of the pontine reticular formation (see Fig. 49). This "nucleus" contributes fibers to a descending reticulospinal tract, which is involved in motor control and plays a major role in the regulation of muscle tone (discussed with Figs. 44 and 45).

The fourth ventricle has become quite wide at this level. At its edges are found the *superior cerebellar peduncles,* exiting from the cerebellum and heading toward the midbrain (red nucleus) and thalamus. The thin sheet of white matter that connects these peduncles is called the *superior medullary velum* (see Fig. 46). These peduncles and the superior medullary velum can be located in a specimen showing the dorsal view of the isolated brain stem (such as the one shown in Fig. 22). These two structures would be found just below the inferior collicular and the exiting fibers of CN IV.

The cerebellum, which is large at this level, is situated behind the ventricle. The lingula of the cerebellum is again labeled and is seen sometimes actually intruding into the ventricular space.

Note: The suggested colors for coding the various nuclei and tracts are indicated in parentheses beside the labeled structures. Please refer to the front of this book (p. ix) for the color coding.

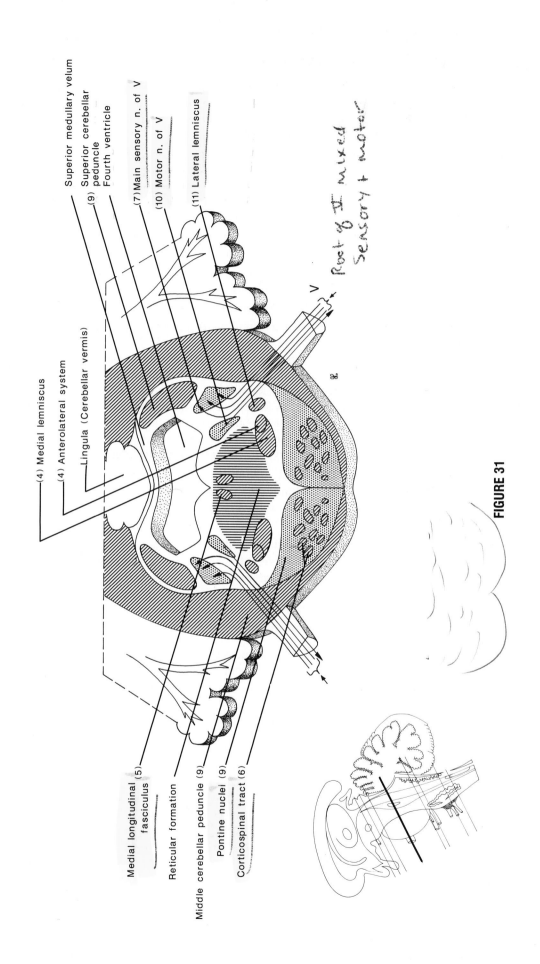

Medial longitudinal (5)
fasciculus

Reticular formation

Middle cerebellar peduncle (9)

Pontine nuclei (9)

Corticospinal tract (6)

(4) Medial lemniscus

(4) Anterolateral system

Lingula (Cerebellar vermis)

Superior medullary velum

(9) Superior cerebellar peduncle

Fourth ventricle

(7) Main sensory n. of V

(10) Motor n. of V

(11) Lateral lemniscus

Root of Ⅴ mixed
Sensory + motor

FIGURE 31

FIGURE 32

Lower Pontine Cross Section (B5)

This cross section of the brain stem including CN V, CN VI, CN VII, and CN VIII is complex because of the number of nuclei related to the cranial nerves located in the tegmental portion at this level. Anteriorly, the pontine nuclei have all but disappeared, and the fiber bundles are likely exclusively corticospinal.

CRANIAL NERVE V.   Some of the fibers of the trigeminal nerve that entered at the mid-pontine level descend into the lower pons, continue through the medulla, and reach the upper level of the spinal cord (see Figs. 24 and 47). This pathway, carrying mainly pain and temperature fibers, is the *descending tract* of V, also called the *spinal tract* of V because it reaches to the level of the spinal cord. Medial to this tract, along its full extent, is a corresponding nucleus, which is called by the same name. Fibers synapse in this nucleus and then ascend (see Figs. 38 and 47).

CRANIAL NERVE VI.   The abducens nucleus is a somatic motor nucleus and is located (as expected) in front of the ventricular system. The MLF, also as usual, is found just anteriorly. The exiting fibers of CN VI are also seen at this level (see Fig. 21).

CRANIAL NERVE VII.   The facial nerve nucleus is located in the ventrolateral portion of the tegmentum, where the branchiomotor nucleus is supposed to be located. Unfortunately, the motor cells are not often seen in most sections, possibly because of the plane of the section or because the cells are intermixed with many others in this region. (The parasympathetic portion of this nucleus is rarely identifiable.)

As explained, the fibers of CN VII form an internal loop (see Fig. 48). It is common to see only parts of the course of this nerve on any one section through this level of the pons, and one must know the course of the nerve to be able to identify it. The diagram is drawn as though the whole course of this nerve is present in a single section.

CRANIAL NERVE VIII: COCHLEAR DIVISION.   The two distinct parts at this level are the crossing fibers, which form the *trapezoid body* (see Fig. 39), and the *superior olivary complex* (shown in the inset), which subserves the function of sound localization (discussed with Fig. 39).

CRANIAL NERVE VIII: VESTIBULAR DIVISION.   The *lateral vestibular nucleus*, with its giant cells, is located at this level at the lateral edge of the fourth ventricle. These large neurons do not form a compact nuclear mass but are dispersed throughout the nuclear area. The *medial vestibular nucleus* is also present at this level, an extension from the medullary region. There is also a small *superior vestibular nucleus* in this region, but it is generally difficult to identify.

The tegmentum of the pons also includes the ascending sensory tracts and the reticular formation. The medial lemniscus is often somewhat obscured by the fibers of the trapezoid body. It is situated close to the midline but has changed its orientation from that seen in the medullary region (e.g., see Fig. 34; see also Fig. 47). The anterolateral system is too small to be identified, but knowledge of its location is important because of lesions that occur in this area. The nuclei of the reticular formation include the *caudal portion* of the pontine reticular formation, which also contributes to the pontine reticulospinal tract (see Fig. 44).

The fourth ventricle is large but often seems smaller because the lobule of the cerebellar vermis, called the *nodulus* (part of the flocculonodular lobe; see Fig. 58), impinges on its space.

The *intracerebellar* (also called the deep cerebellar) *nuclei* also are located at this cross-sectional level. They are found within the white matter of the cerebellum. (These nuclei are discussed with Fig. 60.) Usually only the most lateral and the largest nucleus, the *dentate,* can be identified in the sections.

The lowermost part of the middle cerebellar peduncle can still be identified at this level. Also present is the *inferior cerebellar peduncle,* which enters the cerebellum at a lower level; it is found more internally within the cerebellum as it becomes "covered over" by the fibers of the middle cerebellar peduncle.

Note: The suggested colors for coding the various nuclei and tracts are indicated in parentheses beside the labeled structures. Refer to page ix for the color coding.

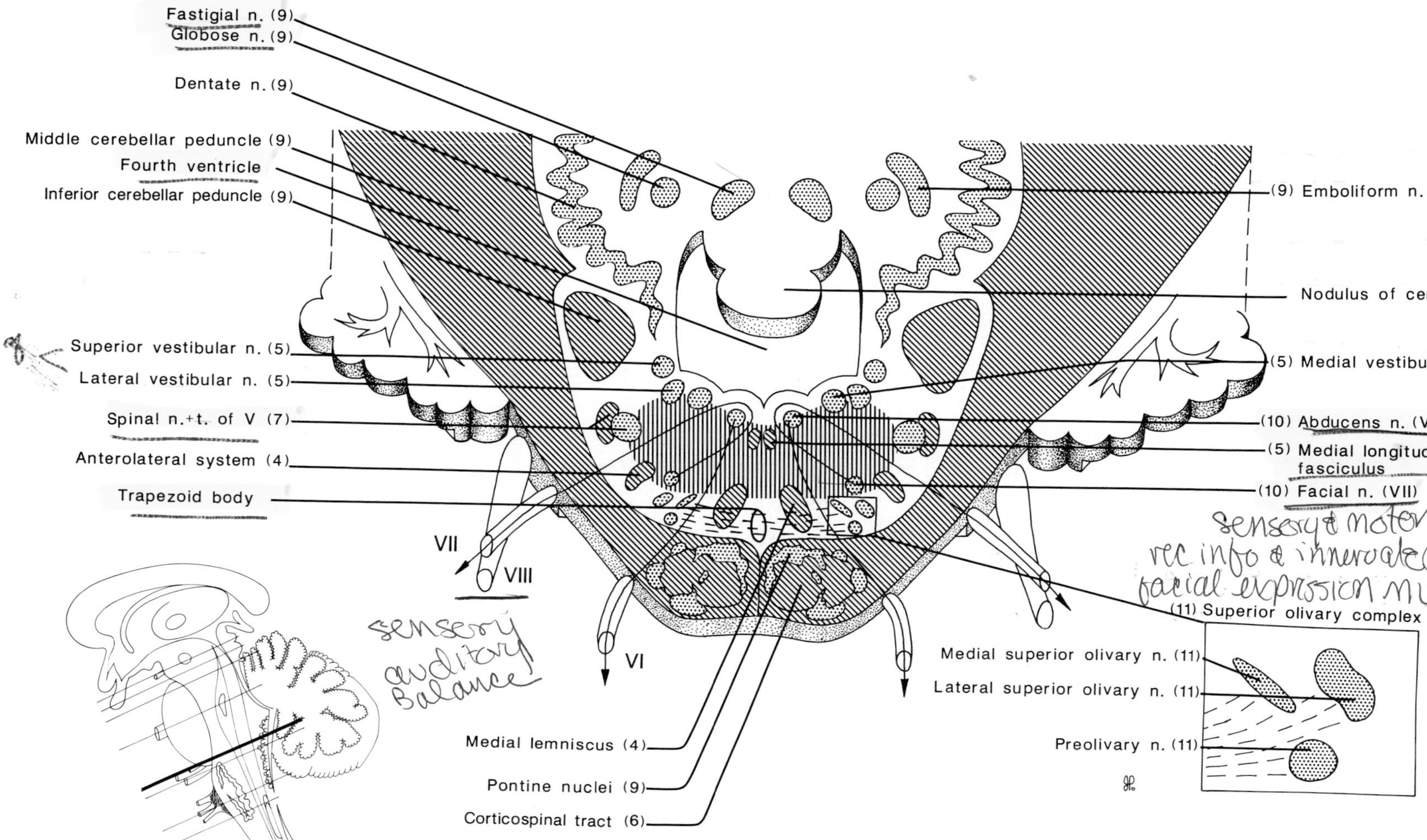

FIGURE 32

Fastigial n. (9)
Globose n. (9)
Dentate n. (9)
Middle cerebellar peduncle (9)
Fourth ventricle
Inferior cerebellar peduncle (9)
Superior vestibular n. (5)
Lateral vestibular n. (5)
Spinal n.+t. of V (7)
Anterolateral system (4)
Trapezoid body

(9) Emboliform n.
Nodulus of cerebellum
(5) Medial vestibular n.
(10) Abducens n. (VI)
(5) Medial longitudinal fasciculus
(10) Facial n. (VII)

Medial superior olivary n. (11)
Lateral superior olivary n. (11)
Preolivary n. (11)
(11) Superior olivary complex

Medial lemniscus (4)
Pontine nuclei (9)
Corticospinal tract (6)

VI
VIII
VII

handwritten annotations:

nuclei of II

motor to rec. info & innervate lat rectus eye muscle

sensory & motor — facial expression muscles

sensory trigeminal

81

PART B–IV

THE MEDULLA (Figures 33–35)

The medulla has a different appearance from the midbrain and pons because of the presence of two distinct structures—the inferior olivary nucleus and the pyramids.

The *inferior olivary nucleus* (also known as the inferior olive) is a prominent nuclear structure that has a distinct scalloped profile when seen in cross section. It is so large that it forms a prominent bulge on the lateral surface of the medulla. Its fibers are distributed to the cerebellum (discussed with Fig. 61).

The *pyramids* are an elevated pair of structures located on either side of the midline. They contain the corticospinal fibers that have descended through the cerebral peduncles of the midbrain, and the pontine region, and that now emerge as a distinct bundle (see Fig. 41). This tract is often called the *pyramidal tract*. Most of its fibers cross (decussate) at the lowermost part of the medulla (see Fig. 48).

The area of the medulla that contains the inferior olivary nucleus, the cranial nerve nuclei, and the nuclei of the reticular formation is the *tegmentum*. Cranial nerves VIII, IX, X, the cranial part of XI, and XII are attached to the medulla and have their nuclei here. The most prominent nucleus of the reticular formation in this region has very large cells and is called the *nucleus gigantocellularis* (see Fig. 49).

Also included in the tegmentum are the various tracts. The ascending fibers include the large bundle, the medial lemniscus, that carries discriminative touch sensation from the body (see Fig. 36). The smaller tract, the anterolateral system, which carries pain and temperature information from the body, is more difficult to recognize. The spinal (descending) tract of V, with its nucleus, conveying pain and temperature from the face and teeth, is also found throughout the medulla (see Fig. 47). One of the most important sensory systems in the medulla is the *solitary nucleus and tract*, which subserve both taste and visceral afferents (discussed with Fig. 24). The MLF is still a distinct tract in its usual location.

The fourth ventricle lies behind the tegmentum, separating the medulla from the cerebellum. It begins to taper and becomes quite narrow in the lowest part of the medulla (see Fig. 46); eventually, it is continuous with the central canal of the spinal cord (see Fig. 10A). The roof of this part of the ventricle has choroid plexus (see Fig. 27). Cerebrospinal fluid escapes from the fourth ventricle through the various foramina located here and flows into the subarachnoid space (see Figs. 10A and 10B).

The medulla is represented by three sections—the upper, mid, and lower medulla:

- The uppermost section typically includes CN VIII (both parts) and its nuclei.
- The section through the middle of the medulla is at the midolivary level and includes the nuclei of CN IX, CN X, and CN XII.
- The lowermost section is at the level of the dorsal column nuclei, the nuclei gracilis and cuneatus, and the decussating fibers of the medial lemniscus.

Lesions in this area of the brain stem are not uncommon. The midline area is supplied by branches from the vertebral artery (see Fig. 20). The structures included in this territory are the corticospinal fibers, the medial lemniscus, and the hypoglossal nerve and nucleus. The lateral portion is supplied by the posterior inferior cerebellar artery, a branch of the vertebral artery (see Fig. 4), often called PICA by neuroradiologists. For an unknown reason, this artery is apparently prone to infarction. Included in its territory are the nuclei and fibers of CN IX and CN X, the descending trigeminal nucleus and tract, fibers of the anterolateral system, and the solitary nucleus and tract, as well as descending autonomic fibers. The whole clinical picture is called the *lateral medullary syndrome*.

It is instructive for a student to work out the clinical symptoms that would be seen when a vascular lesion affects each of these branches. Interruption of the descending autonomic fibers gives rise to a clinical condition called *Horner's syndrome*. In this syndrome, there is loss of the autonomic sympathetic supply to one side of the face, ipsilaterally. This leads to drooping of the upper eyelid, dry skin, and constriction of the pupil. The pupillary change is due to the competing influences of the parasympathetic fibers (from the Edinger-Westphal nucleus), which are still intact. Other lesions can also give rise to Horner's syndrome.

FIGURE 33   # Upper Medullary Cross Section (B6)

This cross section of the brain stem through CN VIII has the characteristic features of the medullary region—namely, the pyramids anteriorly with some remaining parts of the inferior olivary nucleus situated just behind.

The medial lemniscus is the most prominent ascending tract throughout the medulla. The tracts are oriented in the anteroposterior (ventrodorsal) direction, just behind the pyramids (see Fig. 47). Dorsal to the tracts, also along the midline, are the paired tracts of the MLF, situated in front of the fourth ventricle. The anterolateral tract lies dorsal to the olive, although it is not of sufficient size to be clearly identified. Both the medial lemniscus and the anterolateral system are carrying fibers from the other side of the body at this level.

CN VIII enters the medulla at its uppermost level, at the cerebellopontine angle, passing over the inferior cerebellar peduncle. The nerve has two nuclei along its course, the *ventral* and *dorsal cochlear nuclei*. The auditory fibers synapse in these nuclei and then go on to the superior olivary complex in the lower pons region. The crossing fibers are seen in the lowermost pontine region as the trapezoid body (see Figs. 32 and 47).

The vestibular part of CN VIII is represented at this level by two nuclei, the *medial* and *inferior vestibular nuclei*. Both these nuclei lie in the same position as the vestibular nuclei in the pontine section, adjacent to the lateral edge of the fourth ventricle. The inferior vestibular nucleus is distinct because of the many axon bundles that course through it. These vestibular nuclei contribute fibers to the MLF (discussed with Fig. 51).

A nucleus that is seen for the first time is found at this level—the *solitary nucleus,* surrounding a tract of the same name. This nucleus is the synaptic station for incoming taste fibers and for visceral afferents entering with CN IX and CN X. The solitary nucleus and tract are situated just anterior to the vestibular nuclei. The spinal trigeminal nucleus and tract are found in a more lateral location, adjacent to these structures. The core area of the tegmentum is occupied by the cells of the reticular formation.

The other prominent tract in the medullary region is the *inferior cerebellar peduncle* (see Fig. 21). This tract conveys fibers to the cerebellum, both from the spinal cord and the medulla, particularly from the inferior olivary nucleus (see Fig. 61).

The fourth ventricle is still quite large at this level. Its roof has choroid plexus. Behind the ventricle is the cerebellum, with the vermis (midline) portion; the lateral lobule that is present at this juncture is the *cerebellar tonsil* (see Figs. 21 and 59).

Note: The suggested colors for coding the various nuclei and tracts are indicated in parentheses beside the labeled structures. Please refer to the front of this book (p. ix) for the color coding.

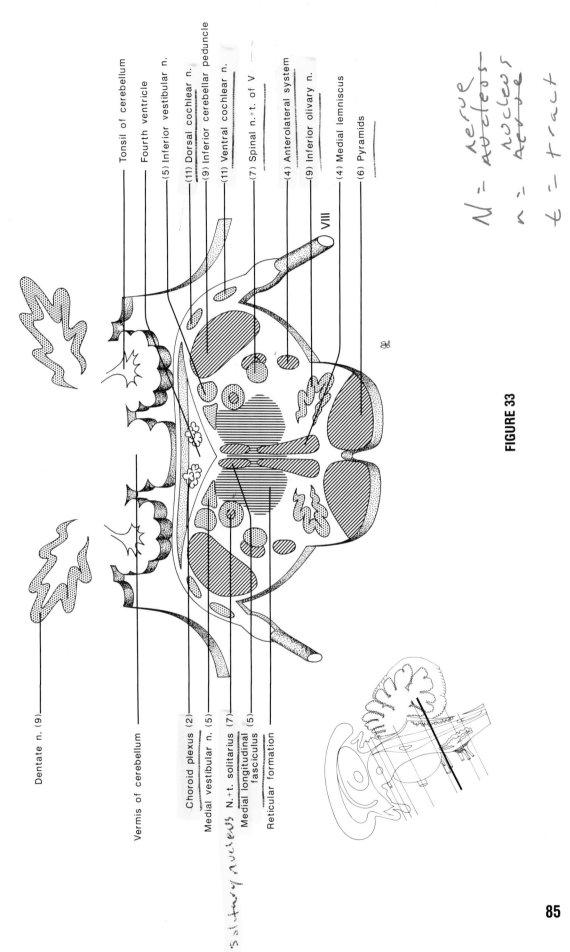

Dentate n. (9)

Vermis of cerebellum

Choroid plexus (2)

Medial vestibular n. (5)

solitary nucleus N.+t. solitarius (7)

Medial longitudinal fasciculus (5)

Reticular formation

Tonsil of cerebellum

Fourth ventricle

(5) Inferior vestibular n.

(11) Dorsal cochlear n.

(9) Inferior cerebellar peduncle

(11) Ventral cochlear n.

(7) Spinal n.+t. of V

(4) Anterolateral system

(9) Inferior olivary n.

(4) Medial lemniscus

(6) Pyramids

VIII

N = nerve nucleus
n = nucleus nerve
t = tract

FIGURE 33

85

FIGURE 34   # Midmedullary Cross Section (B7)

This cross section of the brain stem through the midmedulla is a classic level for descriptive purposes. The inferior olive and pyramids are easily recognized. CN IX, CN X, and CN XII are attached to the medulla at this level with the many nuclei associated with these nerves.

The hypoglossal nucleus (CN XII) is a somatic motor nucleus that occupies the same location—near the midline and in front of the ventricle—as the nuclei of CN III, CN IV, and CN VI. The fibers of CN XII exit anteriorly, between the pyramid and the olive (see Figs. 21 and 23). The MLF lies in front of the nucleus of CN XII, and the medial lemniscus lies in front of that, both situated adjacent to the midline. Lesions of the brain stem in this region (e.g., vascular) may involve this group of structures—namely, the pyramids, the medial lemniscus, and CN XII. The student should try to work out the clinical deficits that would be found following a lesion of this nature (on the left side only).

The other ascending sensory systems are found in the lateral aspect of the medulla. The fibers of the anterolateral system are situated dorsal to the olive. The descending nucleus and tract of the trigeminal system have the same location in the lateral aspect of the tegmentum. Therefore, a lesion here (e.g., occlusion of the posterior inferior cerebellar artery) produces a different pattern of sensory loss (as discussed earlier).

CN IX and CN X are attached at the lateral aspect of the medulla (see Fig. 46). Their efferent fibers are derived from two nuclei—the *dorsal motor nucleus,* which is parasympathetic, and the *nucleus ambiguus,* which is branchiomotor (see Fig. 23). The dorsal motor nucleus lies adjacent to the fourth ventricle just lateral to the nucleus of CN XII. The nucleus ambiguus lies dorsal to the olivary nucleus. In a single cross section, only a few cells of this nucleus are usually seen, making the identification of this nucleus difficult (i.e., "ambiguous") in actual sections. The taste and visceral afferents carried in these nerves synapse in the solitary nucleus, which is located in the posterior aspect of the tegmentum.

The other nuclei in this lateral region of the medulla are sometimes difficult to sort out. The lowermost portions of the inferior and medial vestibular nuclei may still be present at this level. In some sections, the *accessory cuneate nucleus* may be found. This nucleus is a relay for some of the cerebellar afferents from the upper extremity. The fibers then go to the cerebellum through the inferior cerebellar peduncle, which is found along the dorsal margin of the medulla (see Fig. 61).

The reticular formation occupies the central core of the tegmentum, as usual. There are some large cells present at this level, and these are said to form a "nucleus," the *nucleus gigantocellularis,* in this part of the reticular formation (see Fig. 49). These cells give rise to a descending tract (see Fig. 45).

The fourth ventricle is still a rather large space behind the tegmentum, with the choroid plexus attached to its roof (in this area). These structures often are absent in cross sections taken at this level, and the ventricle appears "open." There is no cerebellar tissue posteriorly since the section is below the level of the cerebellum (see the schematic diagram accompanying this figure).

Note: The suggested colors for coding the various nuclei and tracts are indicated in parentheses beside the labeled structures. Please refer to the front of this book (p. ix) for the color coding.

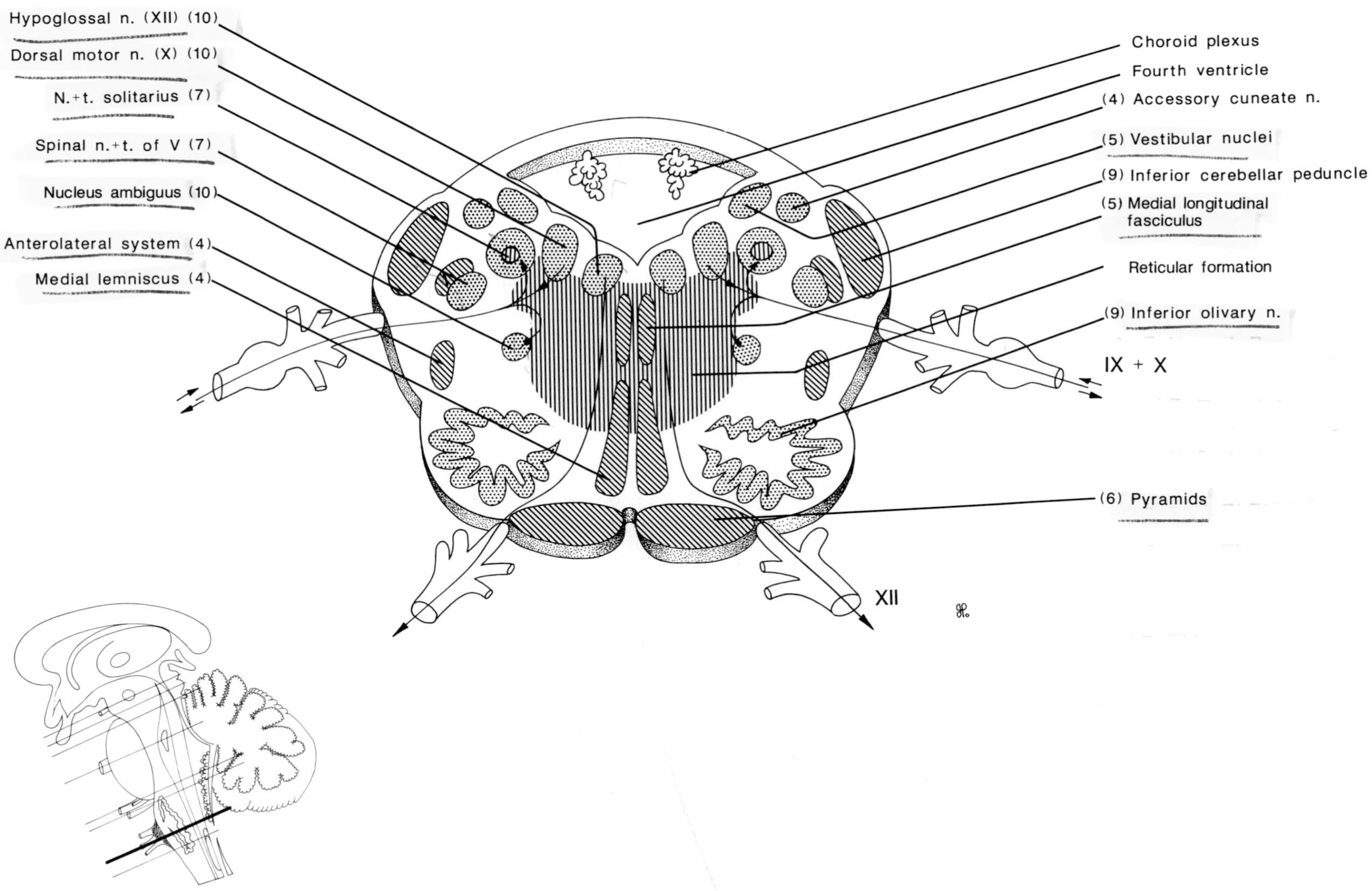

Hypoglossal n. (XII) (10)
Dorsal motor n. (X) (10)
N.+t. solitarius (7)
Spinal n.+t. of V (7)
Nucleus ambiguus (10)
Anterolateral system (4)
Medial lemniscus (4)

Choroid plexus
Fourth ventricle
(4) Accessory cuneate n.
(5) Vestibular nuclei
(9) Inferior cerebellar peduncle
(5) Medial longitudinal fasciculus
Reticular formation
(9) Inferior olivary n.

IX + X

XII

(6) Pyramids

FIGURE 34

FIGURE 35   # Lower Medullary Cross Section (B8)

This is a cross section of the brain stem through the dorsal column nuclei. The medulla seems significantly smaller at this level, approaching the size of the spinal cord below. This section is still easily recognized as medullary because of the presence of the pyramids and the inferior olivary nucleus.

The dorsal aspect of the medullary tegmentum is occupied by two large nuclei—the *nucleus cuneatus* (lateral) and the *nucleus gracilis* (more medial) (see Fig. 46). These nuclei are the synaptic terminations of the tracts of the same name that have ascended the spinal cord (see Fig. 47). The fibers relay here and then move anteriorly to form the medial lemniscus. In so doing, they pass through the tegmentum and are seen as a stream of axons called the *internal arcuate fibers*. These axons actually cross the midline (decussate) to form the *medial lemniscus* of the other side. At this level, the medial lemniscus is situated between the olivary nuclei and dorsal to the pyramids, and is oriented anteroposteriorly.

The nuclei of CN X and CN XII are present as before, as is the descending nucleus and tract of V. (CN XI is discussed with Fig. 48.) The MLF and anterolateral fibers are in the same position. The solitary tract and nucleus are also still found in the same location. The internal arcuate fibers may obscure the exact localization of the nucleus ambiguus. Finally, the reticular formation is still present.

Cross sections through the lowermost part of the medulla may include the decussating corticospinal fibers—that is, the pyramidal decussation (seen in Fig. 48). This would therefore alter significantly what would be seen in the actual cross section.

Posteriorly, the fourth ventricle is tapering down in size, giving a V-shaped appearance to the dorsal aspect of the medulla (see Fig. 46). The ventricle roof is commonly absent at this level, which is probably accounted for by the presence of the foramen of Magendie, where the cerebrospinal fluid escapes from the ventricular system into the subarachnoid space (see Fig. 10A). Posterior to this area is the *cerebellomedullary cistern*, otherwise known as the *cisterna magna* (see Fig. 7, not labeled).

One special nucleus is found in the floor of the ventricle at this level, the *area postrema* (see Fig. 46, not labeled). This forms a little bulge that can be appreciated on some cross sections. The nucleus is part of the system that controls vomiting, and it is often referred to as the vomiting center. This region lacks a blood–brain barrier, allowing this particular nucleus to be exposed directly to whatever is circulating in the blood stream.

Note: The suggested colors for coding the various nuclei and tracts are indicated in parentheses beside the labeled structures. Please refer to the front of this book (p. ix) for the color coding.

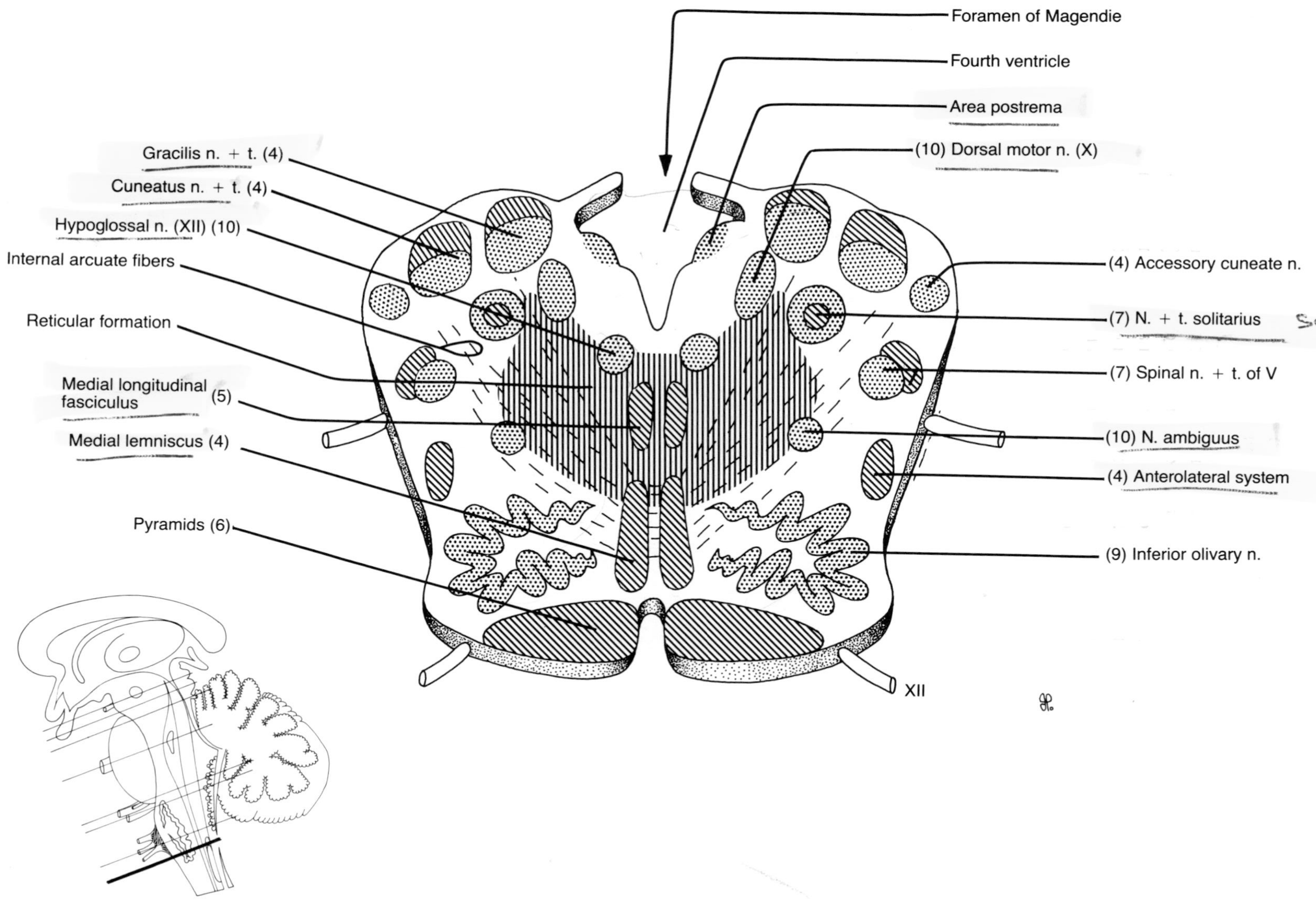

Foramen of Magendie

Fourth ventricle

Area postrema

(10) Dorsal motor n. (X)

(4) Accessory cuneate n.

(7) N. + t. solitarius   Solitary

(7) Spinal n. + t. of V

(10) N. ambiguus

(4) Anterolateral system

(9) Inferior olivary n.

XII

Gracilis n. + t. (4)

Cuneatus n. + t. (4)

Hypoglossal n. (XII) (10)

Internal arcuate fibers

Reticular formation

Medial longitudinal fasciculus (5)

Medial lemniscus (4)

Pyramids (6)

FIGURE 35

89

Pathways of the Central Nervous System (Figures 36–51)

INTRODUCTION

One of the most important aspects of the complexity of our central nervous system (CNS) is communication of one part of the CNS with other parts. The various portions of the CNS communicate with one another by axons of one cell group that connect to the cells and dendrites of another cell group or nucleus. These axons usually run together, forming a distinct bundle of fibers, called a *tract* or *pathway* (or *funiculus*). An example of this is the various pathways linking cortical areas with one another (see Figs. 9A and 9B). Along their way, these axons may distribute information to several other parts of the CNS by means of axon collaterals.

Generally speaking, the older axon systems are thinly myelinated or unmyelinated, with a slow rate of conduction. In general, these pathways consist of fibers–synapses–fibers, creating a multisynaptic chain with many opportunities for spreading the information, but making transmission slow and insecure. The newer pathways that have evolved have axons that are more thickly myelinated and that conduct more rapidly. These form rather direct connections with few, if any, collaterals. The newer pathways transfer information more securely and are more specialized functionally.

This section considers the tracts or pathways carrying sensory information from the periphery into the CNS, and the pathways underlying motor control. The sensory (afferent) tracts begin in the periphery, either in the spinal cord (see Fig. 65) or brain stem, and ascend. The motor (efferent) tracts are more complicated since some begin in the cortex and others in the brain stem. They descend to influence the cranial nerve nuclei and proceed through the spinal cord to the anterior horn cells, the alpha motor neurons (see Fig. 64).

The sensory tracts are also called the *ascending pathways* because they are conveying information upward toward the thalamus and the cortex. Four ascending tracts will be shown:

> *Dorsal column-medial lemniscus pathway*—for the somatosensory sensations of discriminative touch, joint position, and vibration from the body
> *Anterolateral system*—carries pain and temperature, and some less discriminative forms of skin sensations from the body (formerly called the lateral spinothalamic and ventral spinothalamic tracts, respectively)
> *Trigeminal pathways*—carry sensations from the face area (including discriminative touch, pain, and temperature)
> *Auditory pathway*—for the sense of hearing

These tracts relay in the thalamus before going on to the cerebral cortex (see Section D).

The motor tracts are called *descending* because they commence in the cortex or brain stem and influence motor cells lower in the neuraxis, either in the brain stem or spinal cord. These motor neurons are called the *lower motor neurons,* functionally speaking. The neurons giving rise to these pathways are collectively called the *upper motor neurons.* Since all of the descending influences converge on the lower motor neurons, these neurons have also been called, in a functional sense, the *final common pathway*. There are a number of descending tracts or pathways:

> *Corticospinal and corticobulbar tracts:* The corticospinal tract is a relatively new tract and one of the most important for voluntary motor control. Fibers that go to the cranial nerve and other brain stem nuclei form the corticobulbar pathway.
>
> *Rubrospinal tract:* The red nucleus of the midbrain gives rise to the rubrospinal tract.
>
> *Lateral vestibulospinal tract:* The lateral vestibular nucleus of the pons gives rise to the lateral vestibulospinal tract. Other descending vestibular influences join with another tract known as the medial longitudinal fasciculus.
>
> *Reticulospinal tracts:* Two tracts descend from the reticular formation—one from the pontine region, the medial reticulospinal tract, and one from the medulla, the lateral reticulospinal tract.

The tracts will be presented in two ways. On the left side of the page is a schematic diagram of the CNS, showing the spinal cord, the brain stem, and the forebrain. The internal capsule is shown as the area between the diencephalon and the basal ganglia. This diagram will be used to convey the overall system, particularly at what level the fibers cross (decussate) in the CNS. This will assist the student in correlating the anatomy of the pathway with the clinical findings.

On the right side of the page are a series of cross sections through the brain stem and spinal cord. The brain stem sections are the same as those shown in Section B of the *Atlas*. The precise cross section is indicated in the coding used in the headings with the figure number on the page with the text (e.g., B1 refers to the diagram of the midbrain, Fig. 28). (The student may also refer to Figs. 26 and 27 for an orientation to the level of the cross section.) The exact position of the tract within the brain stem or spinal cord is indicated (in black), on the other side, in the cross sections.

The spinal cord cross sections are shown in Section F of the *Atlas*. Level C8 refers to the cervical level of the spinal cord at the eighth segmental level. Level L3 is the third lumbar segment of the spinal cord (not the vertebral level). The position of the various tracts, both ascending and descending, is found in Figure 65.

The last part of this section of the *Atlas* consists of several diagrams specifically illustrating the various pathways that traverse the brain stem. The aim is to present the various sensory pathways in a single diagram; the same is done for the motor tracts. Other special pathways are also discussed. These are all presented from a somewhat different perspective and have been placed separately.

Note to the student: It is recommended that the tracts in Parts C-I and C-II be colored by the student. The visual effect of this simple activity is the creation of an actual pathway. The addition of color visually unites the sections and creates the image of a distinct bundle of fibers coursing within the CNS. Please refer to the front of this book (p. ix) for the suggested color coding.

PART C–I

ASCENDING TRACTS (Figures 36–39)

FIGURE 36   ## Dorsal Column-Medial Lemniscus Pathway

This sensory pathway carries the following modalities from the body: discriminative touch sensation, joint position, and the somewhat artificial "sense" of vibration. In the periphery, the sensory receptors are highly specialized and the fibers are thickly myelinated. The neurons in the dorsal root ganglia are large. Discriminative touch sensation can be tested by asking the patient to identify objects placed in the hand (with the eyes closed); joint position is tested by moving a joint and asking the patient to report the direction of the movement (again with the eyes closed); vibration is tested by placing a tuning fork that has been set into motion onto a bony prominence (e.g., the wrist, the ankle).

The axons enter the spinal cord and ascend, after giving off local collaterals that form the basis of various reflexes. Fibers entering below the level of about T6 form the *fasciculus* (another word for tract) *gracilis;* those entering above T6, particularly those from the upper limb, form the *fasciculus cuneatus,* which is more laterally placed (see Fig. 65). These tracts, together called the *dorsal column,* ascend the spinal cord in the dorsal area and form their first synapse in the lowermost brain stem, in the nuclei that have the same names—the *nuclei gracilis* and *cuneatus* (see Figs. 46 and 47). The fibers of this pathway are well myelinated.

Many axons emanate from the neurons of these two nuclei and course ventromedially within the tegmentum of the lower medulla; these can be recognized at this level and are called the *internal arcuate fibers.* These axons cross the midline and then group together to form the *medial lemniscus.* Initially, this tract is located between the inferior olivary nuclei and is oriented in the dorsoventral position. The tract moves somewhat more posteriorly as it ascends in the medulla. In the pons, it changes its orientation to that of a mediolateral position. The tract is somewhat obscured by the crossing fibers of the trapezoid body (auditory fibers) at the lower level of the pons. In the upper part of the pons, the tract moves more laterally. This movement continues in the midbrain, until the fibers of the anterolateral system and trigeminal system course together with the medial lemniscus. (This shifting of position through the brain stem is also shown in Fig. 47.) This pathway does not give off collaterals in the brain stem to the reticular formation.

The medial lemniscus terminates in the *ventral posterolateral (VPL) nucleus* of the thalamus (see Figs. 53 and 54). After synapsing here, fibers enter the *internal capsule,* its posterior limb, and travel to the somatosensory cortex, terminating along the *postcentral gyrus* (see Fig. 54).

Lesions involving this tract result in the loss of the sensory modalities carried in this pathway. A lesion in the spinal cord causes a loss on the same side; after the synapse and the crossing in the lower brain stem, any lesion of the medial lemniscus results in a loss occurring on the opposite side of the body. Lesions occurring in the midbrain and internal capsule often involve the fibers of the trigeminal system as well as the modalities carried in the anterolateral pathway (to be discussed with Figs. 37 and 38). With cortical lesions, the area of the body affected by a lesion is determined by the area of the postcentral gyrus involved. The postcentral gyrus has a representation of the body called the *sensory homunculus.* The face and the hand are represented on the dorsolateral surface (see Fig. 2), with the lower limb represented on the medial aspect of the hemisphere (see Fig. 7).

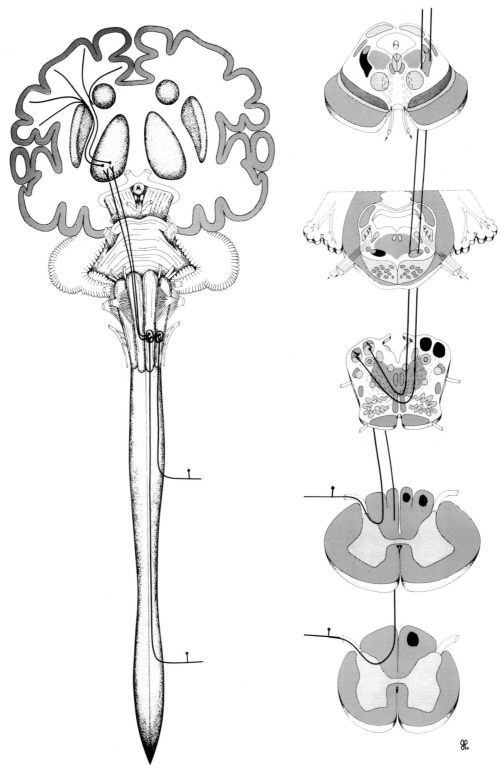

FIGURE 36
With cross-sectional levels B1, B4, B8, C8, L3

FIGURE 37   # Anterolateral System

This sensory pathway carries the modalities of pain and temperature (formerly called the lateral spinothalamic tract) and a form of touch sensation called crude touch (formerly called the anterior spinothalamic tract). Also conveyed in this fiber system are the sensations of itch and tickle, and other forms of sensation (e.g., sensations of a sexual nature). In the periphery, the receptors are usually simply free nerve endings, without any specialization. The axons are poorly myelinated or often unmyelinated, and conduct slowly.

These fibers enter the spinal cord and synapse in the dorsal horn (see Fig. 64). There are many collaterals that are the basis of several protective reflexes. The number of synapses formed is variable and still uncertain, but eventually a neuron is reached that projects its axon up the spinal cord. This axon crosses in the spinal cord, usually two or three segments above the level of entry of the peripheral fibers. These axons now form a tract lying in the anterolateral portion of the white matter of the spinal cord.

The tract ascends in the same position through the brain stem (see Fig. 47), giving off collaterals to the reticular formation. In the medulla, it is situated dorsal to the inferior olivary nucleus. In the pons, it is located lateral to the superior olivary complex. In the uppermost pons and certainly in the midbrain, the fibers join the medial lemniscus. Some of them terminate in the VPL nucleus of the thalamus, and some terminate in the intralaminar nuclei (see Fig. 53).

The axons projecting from the thalamus enter the posterior limb of the internal capsule and are conveyed to several cortical areas, including the postcentral gyrus (also called area SI) and area SII (a secondary sensory area located in the lower portion of the parietal lobe), as well as other cortical regions.

Lesions of this pathway from the point of crossing in the spinal cord upward result in a loss of the modalities of pain and temperature and crude touch on the opposite side of the body. The exact level of the lesion can be accurately ascertained, as the sensation of pain can be simply tested at the bedside by using the end of a pin. (The tester should be aware that this is an uncomfortable and unpleasant sensation for the patient being tested.) In addition, "irritative" lesions of this pathway, whether occurring centrally (including the thalamus) or in the periphery, may result in unusual and unpleasant sensations called *dysesthesia* or *hyperesthesia*.

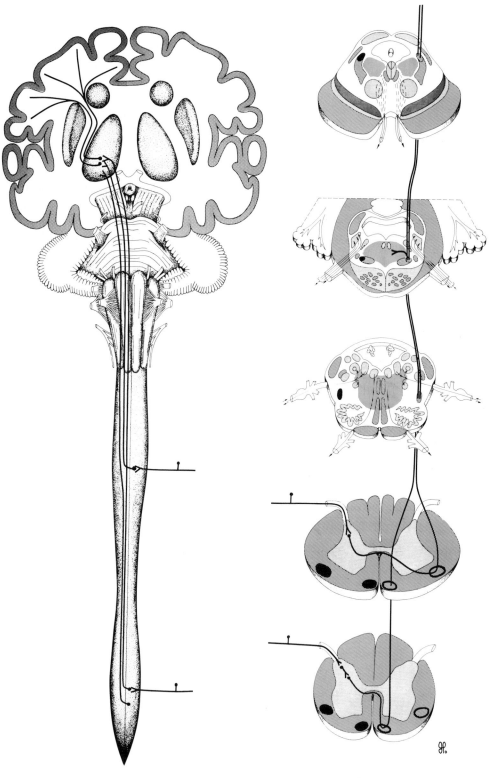

FIGURE 37
With cross-sectional levels B1, B4, B7, C8, L3

FIGURE 38   # Trigeminal System

The sensory fibers come from the face and include all the modalities. The fibers enter the brain stem at the level of the middle cerebellar peduncle (see Fig. 21). Within the CNS, there is a differential handling of the modalities, which allows us to describe the system using the analogy of the dorsal column-medial lemniscus and the anterolateral pathways.

Fibers carrying the sensations of discriminative touch synapse in the principal (main) nucleus of CN V, in the midpons, at the level of entry of the nerve (see Fig. 24). The axons from this nucleus cross and join the medial lemniscus (see Fig. 47). The fibers terminate in the *ventral posteromedial (VPM) nucleus* of the thalamus (see Figs. 53 and 54) and are relayed to the postcentral gyrus through the posterior limb of the internal capsule. The face area is located on the dorsolateral surface and is well represented on the postcentral gyrus. Some sensory input from the midline area of the face ascends on the same side (ipsilaterally), without crossing (not shown here; see Fig. 54).

The fibers carrying the modalities of pain and temperature, including those from the mucous membranes of the mouth and from the teeth, descend within the brain stem. They form a tract that starts at the midpontine level, descends through the medulla, and reaches the upper level of the spinal cord (see Fig. 24). The tract is called the *descending* or *spinal tract of V* (also known as the *spinal trigeminal tract*). Immediately medial to this tract is a nucleus with the same name. The fibers terminate in this nucleus and, after synapsing, cross to the other side and ascend (see Fig. 47). Therefore, these fibers decussate over a wide region, from the pons to the spinal cord, and do not form a compact bundle of crossing fibers. This system gives off collaterals to the reticular formation, just like those of the anterolateral system.

To maintain the comparison, these fibers should join the anterolateral system. The anterolateral pathway, however, joins the medial lemniscus in the pons. Therefore, it is usually said that the trigeminal fibers join the medial lemniscus (see Figs. 47 and 54). The fibers terminate in the VPM nucleus of the thalamus and other thalamic nuclei, and follow the same course as those of the anterolateral system.

There is a particular affliction of the trigeminal nerve called *trigeminal neuralgia*, also known as *tic douloureux*. Sufferers report that they have fleeting sensations of intense pain in the distribution of one of the branches of the trigeminal nerve. The cause of this disorder is sometimes viral and is often unknown. The painful sensations can be brought on by any object touching the skin or even by air currents. As one can imagine, this is an extremely unpleasant and disabling condition. Treatment of this painful affliction, involving drugs or surgery, is fraught with difficulties.

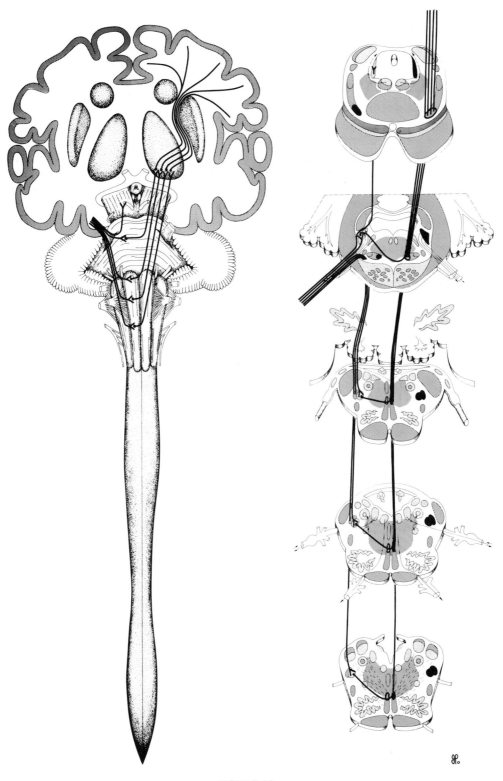

FIGURE 38
With cross-sectional levels B2, B4, B6, B7, B8

FIGURE 39   # Auditory Pathway

The auditory pathway is more complex than the other sensory pathways because there are more nuclei along the way and because the system forms numerous connections across the midline. It also has a unique feature, a feedback pathway from the CNS to the receptor cells in the cochlea.

The fibers from the spiral ganglion, the peripheral ganglion, project to the *dorsal* and *ventral cochlear nuclei.* These nuclei are found along the course of the auditory nerve just as it enters the brain stem at the pontomedullary junction (see Figs. 21, 33, and 47). (In fact, the cochlea is represented three times in these nuclei.) After this, the pathway can follow a number of different routes. In an attempt to make some semblance of order, these will be discussed in sequence, even though an axon may or may not synapse in each of these nuclei.

At the level of the lower pons is the superior olivary complex, which consists of a number of nuclei. Most of the fibers leaving the cochlear nuclei synapse in the *superior olivary complex,* either on the same side or on the opposite side. The fibers cross in the structure known as the *trapezoid body* (see Fig. 47). The main function of the superior olive is sound localization; sound coming from one side will not reach the two ears at the same moment. This differential is processed by the dendrites of the neurons in the superior olive.

Fibers from the superior olivary complex either ascend on the same side or cross in the trapezoid body and ascend on the other side. They form a tract, the *lateral lemniscus,* that begins just above the level of these nuclei (see Fig. 47). It carries the auditory information upward to the inferior colliculus. Nuclei are scattered along the way, interspersed with the lateral lemniscus, and some fibers terminate or relay in these nuclei. The lateral lemnisci are interconnected across the midline throughout the brain stem.

Almost all the axons of the lateral lemniscus terminate in the *inferior colliculus.* These are also interconnected. Next, the fibers leaving the inferior colliculus ascend to the *medial geniculate nucleus* of the thalamus, via the *brachium of the inferior colliculus* (see Figs. 53 and 55). Finally, the axons project via the inferior portion of the internal capsule, the auditory radiation, to the auditory cortex. The gyri that receive the auditory information are found in the superior aspect of the temporal lobe, which is buried in the lateral fissure. The two gyri are known as the *transverse gyri of Heschl* (shown in Fig. 3).

In summary, there are numerous opportunities for synapses along the course of the auditory pathway. The name *lemniscus* is rather unfortunate because this pathway does not transmit in the efficient manner seen in the case of the medial lemniscus. Although the pathway is predominantly a crossed system, there is a significant ipsilateral component. There are also numerous interconnections between the two sides. Therefore, a lesion of the auditory pathway on one side does not lead to a total loss of hearing on the other side.

The auditory pathway has a feedback system from the higher levels to lower levels (e.g., from the inferior colliculus to the superior olivary complex). The final link in this feedback is unique in the mammalian CNS, for it influences the receptor cell itself. This pathway, known as the *olivocochlear bundle,* has its cells of origin in the vicinity of the superior olivary complex. It has both a crossed and an uncrossed component. Its axons reach the hair cells of the cochlea by traveling in CN VIII. This system changes the responsiveness of the peripheral hair cells.

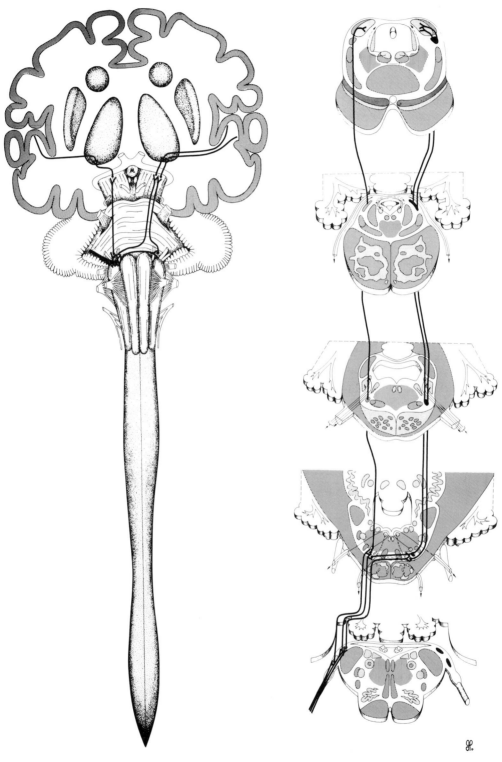

FIGURE 39
With cross-sectional levels B2, B3, B4, B5, B6

PART C–II

DESCENDING TRACTS (Figures 40–45)

FIGURE 40   ## Corticobulbar and Corticopontine Fibers

Fibers descend from the cerebral cortex to all parts of the neuraxis. Many of these fibers are involved in motor control. These axons, part of the so-called projection fibers of the hemispheres, course through the internal capsule (see Fig. 17). Some terminate in the thalamic nuclei; the remainder descend and continue into the cerebral peduncles of the midbrain.

The cerebral peduncle can be divided into three parts—the middle third and the outer and inner thirds (see Fig. 48). The *corticopontine* fibers are found in the inner and outer thirds; the frontopontine fibers are located in the inner third; and fibers from the other lobes are located in the outer third. Most of the fibers terminate in the pontine nuclei, where they synapse. The axons of these pontine nuclei then cross and form the middle cerebellar peduncle (see Fig. 59).

The fibers of the middle third are destined for the brain stem and the spinal cord. The brain stem fibers are called *corticobulbar,* and the spinal fibers *corticospinal.* The corticospinal fibers are discussed with the next diagram.

Corticobulbar fibers are those that go to the cranial nerve nuclei (for motor see Fig. 23), the reticular formation, and other nuclei of the brain stem. According to convention, the cortical motor cells are called the *upper motor neuron* and the motor neurons of the cranial nerves of the brain stem are called the *lower motor neuron.* These motor nuclei are generally innervated by fibers from both sides (i.e., each nucleus receives input from both hemispheres). Therefore, loss of cortical innervation is usually associated with a weakness, not paralysis, of the muscles supplied. There are two exceptions to this rule that are important in the clinical setting.

1   The major exception to this rule is the cortical input to the facial nucleus. In this case, there is a most important difference between the innervation to the upper and lower face. The lower facial muscles receive only a crossed input from the cortex. The nerve supply to the upper facial muscles is derived from both hemispheres. Therefore, a patient with a lesion of the appropriate area of the cortex or of the corticobulbar fibers on one side is able to wrinkle his or her forehead normally on both sides but is unable to show the teeth symmetrically. Because of the marked weakness of the muscles of the lower face, there is a drooping of the lower face on the side opposite the lesion. This also affects the muscle of the cheek (the buccinator muscle) and causes some difficulties with drinking, eating, and chewing (the food gets stuck in the cheek and often has to be manually removed). Often saliva drools on the weakened side.

2   The cortical innervation to the hypoglossal nucleus is not always bilateral. Only some individuals have a predominantly crossed innervation. Therefore, examination of the movements of the tongue does not provide a clear indication of the presence or absence of a lesion of the corticobulbar fibers.

The corticoreticular fibers are extremely important for some voluntary movements and for muscle tone. This indirect pathway is apparently an older pathway for the control of movements, particularly of axial musculature and the proximal joints. (The descending fibers from the reticular formation are shown in Figs. 44, 45, and 49.) Therefore, some voluntary movements can still be performed after destruction of the corticospinal pathway. This pathway is not involved in the fine motor control of the fingers and hand. Destruction of the cortical input to the reticular formation results in a significant change of muscle tone (see Fig. 45).

Cortical fibers probably influence all the brain stem nuclei, with the exception of the lateral vestibular nucleus (see Fig. 43). The cortical input to the sensory nuclei, including the nuclei cuneatus and gracilis, provides some type of feedback; this is likely responsible for sharpening the focus of the input, a psychological phenomenon involved in attention.

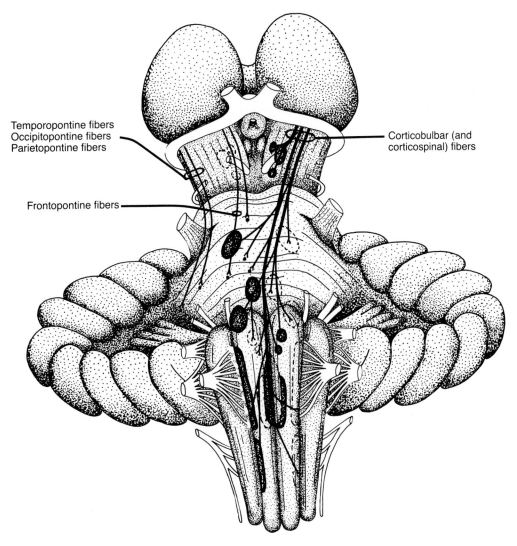

Temporopontine fibers
Occipitopontine fibers
Parietopontine fibers

Frontopontine fibers

Corticobulbar (and
corticospinal) fibers

FIGURE 40

FIGURE 41   # Corticospinal Tract

The corticospinal tract is a direct pathway linking the cortex with the spinal cord. It is one of the newer pathways from the evolutionary point of view (e.g., it is not present in the rat).

Functionally, it is the motor aspects of the corticospinal tract that dominate by influencing the anterior horn cells rather quickly and sometimes directly. This tract is the most important one for voluntary motor movements. Some of these fibers originate in the deeper layers of the precentral gyrus (area 4), whereas others come from other motor areas (e.g., area 6). Some of these fibers, particularly those involved in fine motor movements of the fingers and hands, terminate directly on the anterior horn cells.

Other cells contributing to this system are found in the sensory cortical areas (e.g., the postcentral gyrus). These carry "instructions" from the cortex to the dorsal horn of the spinal cord (its sensory portion; see Fig. 64) that may modify the transmission of sensory information at the spinal cord level. These are similar to the corticobulbar fibers that go to the nuclei gracilis and cuneatus in the lower brain stem.

The axons descend (with the corticobulbar fibers) through the white matter of the hemispheres and go through the posterior limb of the internal capsule (see Fig. 17). They then travel in the midportion of the cerebral peduncles (see Fig. 48) in the midbrain. The corticospinal fibers are found in the pontine region as bundles of axons between the pontine nuclei. These collect in the medulla as a single tract, one on each side of the midline. These fibers now form the structures known as the *pyramids* (see Fig. 21). Hence, the corticospinal pathway is often called the *pyramidal tract*.

At the lowermost part of the medulla, most (90%) of the corticospinal fibers decussate and form the *lateral corticospinal tract* (see Figs. 21 and 48). This tract is located in the lateral portion of the white matter of the spinal cord (see Fig. 65). The lateral corticospinal tract is involved with controlling the individualized movements of our fingers and hands (i.e., the distal limb musculature). These neurons are located in the laterally placed collections of neurons found in the segments giving rise to the brachial plexus (see Figs. 64 and 66). It likely innervates similar neurons in the lower extremity.

Fibers that do not cross in the pyramidal decussation form the *anterior* (or *ventral*) *corticospinal tract*. The ventral pathway is found in the ventral portion of the white matter of the spinal cord (see Fig. 65). Many of these axons cross before terminating, whereas others supply motor neurons on both sides. The ventral pathway is concerned with movements of the axial musculature and proximal limb joints.

Motor control involves the direct (corticospinal) tract, influencing the distal limb musculature, and indirect pathways from the brain stem (with their cortical input), which control the proximal joint movements and axial musculature. Most clinical lesions affect both types of pathways (e.g., a lesion in the internal capsule). Experimentally, after a lesion was placed in the medullary pyramid of monkeys, the animals were capable of almost all movements after 2 to 3 weeks of weakness, but had lost their ability to perform the fine movements of the fingers and hand (on the opposite side); muscle tone remained decreased. This is in comparison with other lesions involving the indirect pathways that lead in time to an increase in tone and reflexes (discussed with Figs. 43 and 45).

There is one abnormal reflex that indicates, in humans, that a lesion has interrupted the corticospinal pathway. The reflex involves stroking the bottom of the foot (a most uncomfortable sensation for most people). Normally, the response involves flexion of the toes, called a *plantar (flexor) response,* and often an attempt to withdraw the limb. After a lesion interrupting the corticospinal pathway, stroking of the bottom of the foot results in an upward movement of the big toe (extension) and a fanning apart of the other toes. The whole response is called a *Babinski sign* and is found almost immediately after any lesion that interrupts the lateral corticospinal pathway, from cortex through to spinal cord. Most interesting, the Babinski "reflex" is present in infants and disappears sometime during the second year of life, concurrent with the myelination that occurs in this pathway.

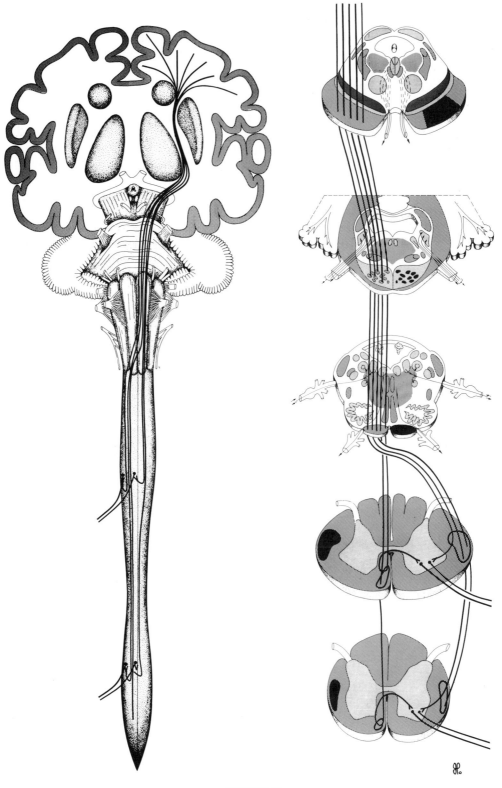

FIGURE 41
With cross-sectional levels B1, B4, B7, C8, L3

FIGURE 42   # Rubrospinal Tract

The motor pathway originates in the red nucleus of the upper midbrain. The cells of origin are large cells located in the ventral part of the nucleus. The red nucleus receives input from the motor areas of the cerebral cortex and from the cerebellum. The cortical input is directly onto the projecting cells, thus forming the two-step pathway from motor cortex to spinal cord.

The rubrospinal tract is also a crossed pathway, with the decussation occurring in the ventral part of the midbrain (see Figs. 48 and 51). The tract descends within the tegmentum (the central part of the brain stem) and is not clearly distinguishable from other fiber systems. The fibers then course in the lateral portion of the white matter of the spinal cord, just anterior to and intermingled with the lateral corticospinal tract (see Fig. 65).

The rubrospinal tract is a well-developed pathway in monkeys. The pathway provides a two-step link from the cortex to the spinal cord. In monkeys, it seems to be involved in flexion movements of the limbs. Stimulation of this tract in cats produces an increase in tone of the flexor muscles.

The functional significance of this pathway in humans is not well known. The number of large cells in the red nucleus in the human is significantly less than that in the monkey. A motor deficit associated with a lesion involving only the red nucleus or only the rubrospinal tract has not been described. Although the rubrospinal pathway may play a role in some flexion movements, it seems that the corticospinal tract predominates in humans.

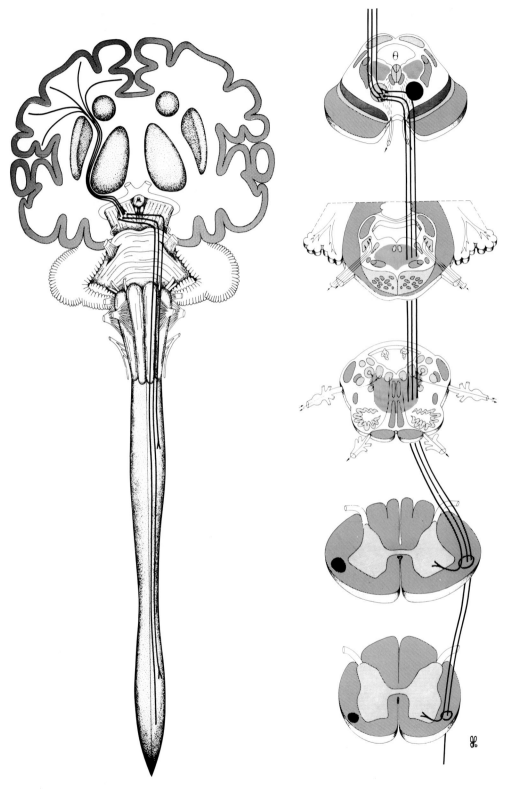

FIGURE 42
With cross-sectional levels B1, B4, B7, C8, L3

FIGURE 43   # Lateral Vestibulospinal Tract

This motor pathway is an important one in that it provides a link between the vestibular influences (i.e., gravity and balance) and the spinal cord. The main function is to provide corrective muscle activity when the body (and head) tilt or change orientation in space.

This tract originates in the *lateral vestibular nucleus,* which is located in the lower pontine region (see Figs. 24 and 51). The nucleus is found at the lateral edge of the fourth ventricle and is characterized by extremely large neurons. (This nucleus is also called *Deiters' nucleus,* and the large neurons are often known by the same name.)

The lateral vestibular nucleus receives its input from the vestibular system and from the cerebellum; there is no cerebral cortical input. This tract descends through the medulla and traverses the entire spinal cord. It does not decussate. In the spinal cord, the tract is positioned anteriorly, just in front of the ventral horn (see Fig. 65). The fibers terminate in the medial portion of the anterior horn—namely, on the motor cells that control the axial musculature.

Functionally, the lateral vestibulospinal pathway increases extensor muscle tone and activates extensor muscles. It is easier to think of these muscles as antigravity muscles in four-legged animals; in humans, one must translate these muscles as the extensors in the lower extremity and the flexors in the upper extremity.

A lesion involving the descending motor fibers in the humans—for example, in the internal capsule—is followed after about 1 week by an increase in muscle tone in the antigravity muscles (*hypertonia*) and an increase in reflex responsiveness in these muscles (*hyperreflexia*). The change in tone, called *spasticity,* and reflexes, is thought to be due in large part to the persistent influence of the vestibulospinal system. Apparently, other systems that have lost their cortical input are no longer activated and are not available to counteract this vestibular influence (discussed with Fig. 45).

OTHER VESTIBULAR CONNECTIONS

The other vestibular nuclei contribute to the medial longitudinal fasciculus (MLF). Some of these fibers descend to the cervical spinal cord, and others ascend to the midbrain. They form part of the interconnecting fiber system that coordinates movements of the eyes and the head and neck with vestibular and visual input. These descending fibers also influence mainly "axial" muscles. This descending pathway is sometimes called the *medial vestibulospinal tract.* (See Fig. 51 for further discussion of other vestibular connections.)

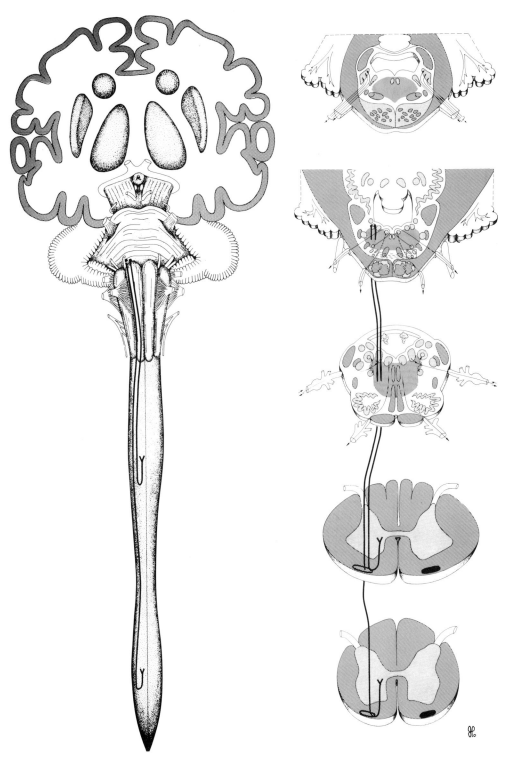

FIGURE 43
With cross-sectional levels B4, B5, B7, C8, L3

Reticulospinal Tracts

As has been noted (see Figs. 25 and 49), the reticular formation is a collection of nuclei that participates in a number of functions, some general (e.g., arousal) and others more specific (e.g., respiratory control). Parts of this system are also involved in voluntary motor movements, forming part of the indirect system of motor control.

The reticular formation receives input from many sources. The input from the cerebral cortex is most important for voluntary control and for the regulation of muscle tone. These axons form part of the *corticobulbar system of fibers*.

There are two pathways from the reticular formation to the spinal cord, one originating in the pontine region and one in the medullary region.

FIGURE 44

Pontine (Medial) Reticulospinal Tract

This tract originates in the pontine reticular formation from two nuclei: the upper one is called the *nucleus reticularis pontis oralis,* and the lower or caudal portion is called the *pontis caudalis.* (These nuclei can be seen in Fig. 49.) It is easier to refer to these as the oral and caudal portions of the pontine reticular nuclei. The tract descends to the spinal cord and is located in the medial portion of the white matter (see Fig. 65). Therefore, this pathway is called the *medial reticulospinal tract.*

Functionally, the action of this pathway is on the extensor muscles, both movements and tone. The area in the pons is known as the *reticular extensor facilitatory area.* The fibers terminate on the anterior horn cells that control the axial muscles. In this way, this system is similar to that of the lateral vestibular nucleus.

Lesions involving the corticobulbar fibers will be discussed with the medullary reticular formation (see Fig. 45).

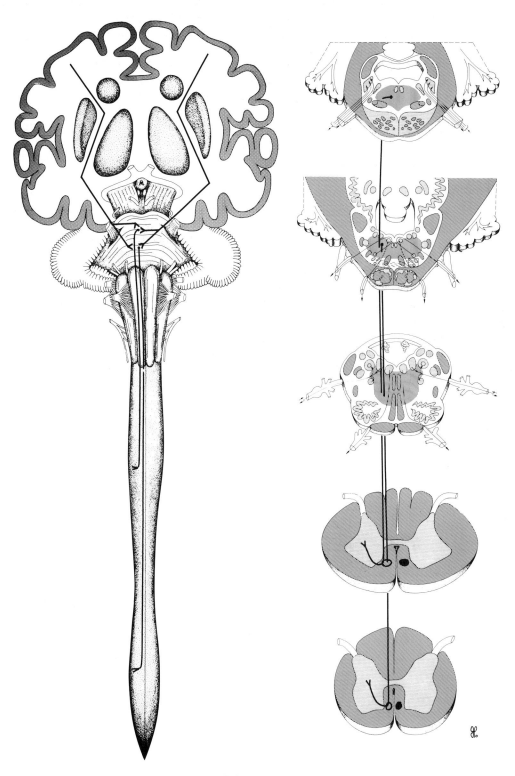

FIGURE 44
With cross-sectional levels B4, B5, B7, C8, L3

FIGURE 45 # Medullary (Lateral) Reticulospinal Tract

This tract originates in the medullary reticular formation, mainly from the nucleus known as the *nucleus gigantocellularis* (see Fig. 49). The tract descends more laterally than the pontine pathway and is named the *lateral reticulospinal tract* (see Fig. 65). Some of the fibers are crossed. The tract lies beside the vestibulospinal pathway.

The medullary reticulospinal tract also has its greatest influence on axial musculature, and its functional contribution has been classified as the *reticular extensor inhibitory area*. In this way, its influence is opposite that of the pontine reticular formation. This area depends for its normal activity on influences coming from the cerebral cortex.

Destruction of the cortical input to the reticular formation results in a significant loss of ongoing activity of the medullary reticular formation, while the pontine reticular formation continues to be active. Therefore, disruption of these descending influences disturbs the balance between the two parts of the reticular formation, with the pontine activity prevailing. This leads to an alteration of muscle tone, with the dominance of the pontine reticulospinal system, plus the ongoing vestibulospinal system. The end result is an increase in the tone and in the reflex responses of the extensor (antigravity) muscles.

This is thought to be the neurophysiologic basis for the increased tone and reflexes that develop after a lesion involving the descending motor pathways above the pontine level in humans. In the clinical setting, this change in reflex responsiveness is called *hyperreflexia* and the change in tone is called *spasticity*. (This is also discussed with Fig. 49.)

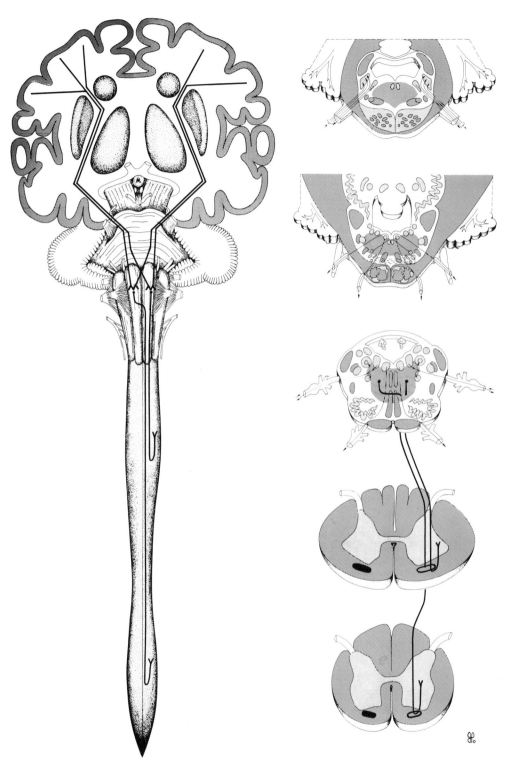

FIGURE 45
With cross-sectional levels B4, B5, B7, C8, L3

PART C–III

BRAIN STEM PATHWAYS (Figures 46–51)

FIGURE 46   ### Brain Stem: Dorsal View

A complete understanding of the brain stem requires assimilating information about the intrinsic nuclei located at different levels, the cranial nerve nuclei, and the various tracts, both ascending (sensory) and descending (motor). It is probably not possible to present all this information in a single diagram. Therefore, a series of diagrams has been developed to help the student understand the complex nature of the brain stem. The series includes:

- the ascending tracts and sensory portions of the cranial nerve nuclei
- the descending tracts and the motor portions of the cranial nerve nuclei
- the reticular formation and its pathways
- pathways involved in integrating eye movements and coordinating visual and vestibular information with movements of the head and neck, the MLF system

The view of the brain stem that has been used for this series of diagrams is an oblique perspective from behind (similar to the view presented in Fig. 22), with the cerebellum removed. An anterior view might have been preferable (see Figs. 21 and 23), but this dorsal perspective seemed more appropriate for the combined visualization of many of the cranial nerve nuclei and the various pathways.

The initial diagram of this series shows the brain stem from this dorsal perspective:

The midbrain is seen with the superior and inferior colliculi (as in Fig. 22). These colliculi form the *quadrigeminal plate,* also called the *tectal plate* or *tectum.* The brachium of the inferior colliculus leads to the *medial geniculate body,* which belongs to the thalamus (see Fig. 55). More anteriorly, in the interior of the midbrain, the *red nucleus* is shown. This view also shows the back edge of the *cerebral peduncle,* the most anterior structure of the midbrain (see Fig. 21). The trochlear nerves (CN IV) emerge at the lower level of the midbrain, below the inferior colliculi (as in Fig. 22).

The dorsal aspect of the pons is represented, with most of the fourth ventricle unroofed. The roof of the upper portion of the fourth ventricle is still preserved and is called the *superior medullary velum.* More important, it contains the *superior cerebellar peduncles* (see Figs. 47 and 63). The floor of the fourth ventricle, as seen from this perspective, has large bumps in its midportion, each called a *facial colliculus,* formed by the fibers of the facial nerve as they go through their internal loop around the abducens nucleus (shown in Fig. 48). Because the cerebellum has been removed, the cut edges of the middle cerebellar peduncles are seen. The trigeminal nerve (CN V) attaches to the brain stem along this peduncle.

The posterior aspect of the medulla is known in traditional sources as the floor of the fourth ventricle. (Some acoustic striae, belonging to CN VIII, are also shown.) The cut edges outline the lower limits of the fourth ventricle. At the lowermost portions of the ventricle are found two large protuberances on either side of the midline. These are the nuclei of the dorsal column pathways, the *nuclei gracilis* and *cuneatus.* The fiber tracts of the same names terminate in these nuclei at the lower level of the medulla (shown in Fig. 47 and seen in cross section in Fig. 35). The nucleus gracilis is located medially, and the lateral one is the nucleus cuneatus. More anteriorly, from this oblique view, are the fibers of the vagus (CN X) and glossopharyngeal (CN IX) nerves, as these emerge from the lateral aspect of the medulla, behind the inferior olive. The inferior cerebellar peduncle (on one side) is also seen as it begins to enter the cerebellum (see Figs. 21 and 61).

A representative cross section of the spinal cord is also shown from this posterior perspective.

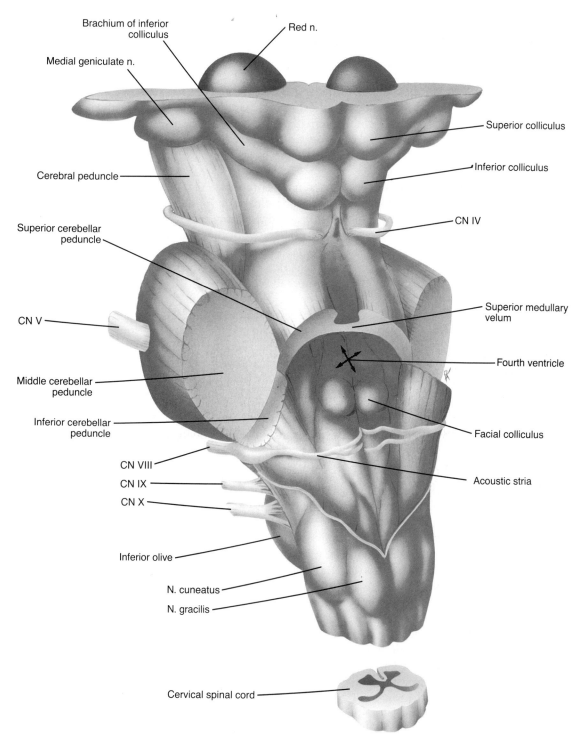

Brachium of inferior colliculus

Medial geniculate n.

Red n.

Cerebral peduncle

Superior colliculus

Inferior colliculus

CN IV

Superior cerebellar peduncle

CN V

Superior medullary velum

Fourth ventricle

Middle cerebellar peduncle

Inferior cerebellar peduncle

Facial colliculus

CN VIII

CN IX

CN X

Acoustic stria

Inferior olive

N. cuneatus

N. gracilis

Cervical spinal cord

FIGURE 46

FIGURE 47   # Ascending Tracts and Sensory Nuclei

This diagramatic presentation of the internal structures of the brain stem is shown from the same perspective as in Fig. 46. The information concerning the various structures will be presented in an abbreviated manner, since most of these have been reviewed in previous sections of the *Atlas*.

The major sensory tracts include the following:

Medial lemniscus (discriminative touch, vibration, and joint position [see Fig. 36]): The dorsal columns of the spinal cord terminate (synapse) in the nuclei gracilis and cuneatus in the lowermost medulla. Axons from these nuclei then cross the midline (decussate) as the internal arcuate fibers (see cross section in Fig. 35), forming a new bundle called the *medial lemniscus*. These fibers ascend through the brain stem and move laterally. There are no collaterals from this pathway to the reticular formation.

Anterolateral system (pain and temperature [see Fig. 37]): This tract ascends from the spinal cord through the brain stem, posterior to the inferior olive (see cross section in Fig. 35). Collaterals from this pathway are given off to the reticular formation, including the periaqueductal gray (not shown here but shown in Fig. 49). At the upper pontine level, this tract becomes associated with the medial lemniscus and the two lie adjacent to each other in the midbrain region. Some of its fibers enter the superior colliculus (not labeled).

Lateral lemniscus (audition [see Fig. 39]): The auditory fibers (CN VIII) enter the brain stem in the lowermost portion of the pons. After the initial synapse in the cochlear nuclei, many of the fibers cross the midline, forming the trapezoid body (see cross section in Fig. 32). Some of the fibers synapse in the superior olivary complex. From this point, the tract known as the *lateral lemniscus* is formed. It terminates in the inferior colliculus. Its continuation, which is not shown in this diagram, is by means of the brachium of the inferior colliculus to the *medial geniculate* (body) *nucleus* (see Figs. 46 and 55).

The sensory cranial nerve nuclei include the following:

Trigeminal nerve (all modalities [see Fig. 38]): The incoming fibers divide, with those for discriminative touch synapsing in the principal nucleus then crossing; these ascend and join with the medial lemniscus. The fibers carrying pain and temperature descend through the pons and medulla as the descending (spinal) trigeminal tract. These fibers then synapse in the adjacent nucleus, the descending (spinal) nucleus of V. Axons from this nucleus cross the midline and ascend, merging with the medial lemniscus at the level of the midbrain (see also Fig. 54).

Facial nerve (sensory afferents and taste): Sensory fibers entering in the facial nerve (CN VII) include some afferents from the ear and taste fibers from the anterior two thirds of the tongue. The sensory afferents join those of the descending nucleus of V. The taste fibers (not shown) synapse in the solitary nucleus (not shown), which lies adjacent to the descending tract and nucleus of V (see Fig. 24; also seen in cross section in Fig. 33) in the medulla.

Glossopharyngeal and vagus nerves (sensory and visceral afferents, and taste): These convey mainly visceral afferents, as well as taste fibers from the posterior one third of the tongue (CN IX) and also the epiglottis region (CN X). These fibers (not shown) synapse in the solitary nucleus. The few sensory fibers from the ear and meninges join with the descending nucleus of V.

The superior cerebellar peduncles are shown, located within the roof of the fourth ventricle, the superior medullary velum. These decussate in the lower midbrain at the inferior collicular level (shown in cross section in Fig. 29), with some fibers terminating in the red nucleus and others continuing on to the thalamus (see Figs. 57 and 63).

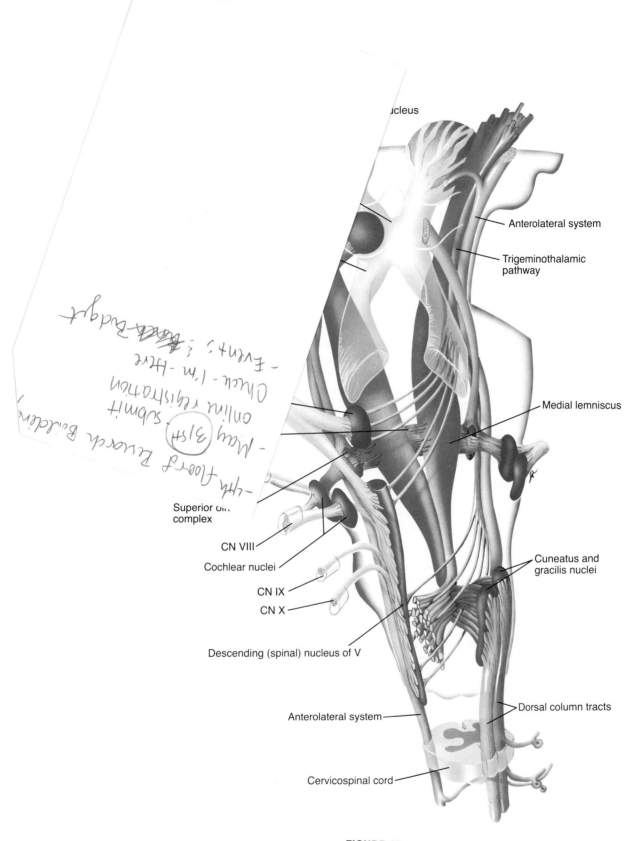

ucleus

Anterolateral system

Trigeminothalamic pathway

Medial lemniscus

Superior ol.
complex

CN VIII

Cochlear nuclei

CN IX

CN X

Cuneatus and gracilis nuclei

Descending (spinal) nucleus of V

Anterolateral system

Dorsal column tracts

Cervicospinal cord

FIGURE 47

FIGURE 48 ## Descending Tracts and Motor Nuclei

Using the somewhat oblique posterior view of the brain stem, various descending tracts are presented, along with those cranial nerve nuclei that have a motor component. Not included is the reticular formation (see Fig. 49) and the related reticulospinal pathways. The pathways associated with the vestibular nuclei, including the MLF and the lateral vestibulospinal tract, are also not included in this diagram (see Fig. 51).

The major motor pathways include the following:

Corticopontine fibers (see Fig. 40): The descending cortical fibers from various parts of the cerebral cortex are found in the outer and inner thirds of the cerebral peduncles. After synapsing in the pontine nuclei (Fig. 31), the fibers cross and project to the cerebellum via the middle cerebellar peduncle.

Corticobulbar fibers (see Fig. 40): These cortical fibers project to the cranial nerve nuclei of the brain stem, to the reticular formation, and to other brain stem nuclei. They descend in the middle third of the cerebral peduncle and are given off at various levels within the brain stem.

Corticospinal tract (see Fig. 41): These fibers also course in the middle third of the cerebral peduncle, then become dispersed in the pontine region (see Fig. 31), between the pontine nuclei, and regroup as a compact bundle in the medulla; here they are frequently called the *pyramidal tract*. At the lowermost part of the medulla (see Fig. 21), most of the fibers decussate to form the lateral corticospinal tract. Some fibers continue ipsilaterally as the anterior (ventral) corticospinal tract.

Rubrospinal tract (see Fig. 42): These fibers, which originate from the lower portion of the red nucleus, decussate in the midbrain region (see Fig. 51) and descend. In the spinal cord, they are located anterior to the lateral corticospinal tract (see Fig. 65).

The cranial nerve nuclei include (see Fig. 23):

Oculomotor (to most extraocular muscles): This large nucleus, located at the level of the superior colliculus, sends its fibers anteriorly; these traverse the medial portion of the red nucleus, before exiting in the interpeduncular fossa (see Fig. 28). The parasympathetic fibers associated with CN III originate from the Edinger-Westphal nucleus.

Trochlear (to the superior oblique muscle): The fibers from this nucleus cross before exiting from the midbrain posteriorly (see Fig. 30). They then wrap around the cerebral peduncles in their course anteriorly (see Figs. 22 and 23).

Trigeminal (to muscles of mastication): The motor fibers pierce the middle cerebellar peduncle as they exit in the pontine region (see Fig. 31).

Abducens (to the lateral rectus muscle): The anterior course of the exiting fibers could not be depicted from this perspective (see Fig. 21).

Facial (to muscles of facial expression): The fibers have an internal loop before exiting (seen in cross section in Fig. 32). The nerve loops over the abducens nucleus, forming a bump called the *facial colliculus* in the floor of the fourth ventricle (see Fig. 46). The nerve of only one side is shown in this illustration.

Glossopharyngeal and vagus (branchiomotor and parasympathetic): The fibers exit behind the inferior olive (see Fig. 23), on the lateral aspect of the medulla. These fibers include those from the nucleus ambiguus (branchiomotor to muscles of the pharynx and larynx) and the parasympathetic fibers from the dorsal motor nucleus of the vagus that supply the structures in the neck, thorax, and abdomen. The fibers of CN XI, the spinal accessory, that originate from the nucleus ambiguus, will join CN X immediately after exiting. (This joining is not shown here.)

Spinal accessory (to neck muscles): The fibers that supply the large muscles of the neck (sternomastoid and trapezius) originate in the upper spinal cord and ascend before exiting from the skull. When referring to the spinal accessory nerve, one usually has in mind only this component.

Hypoglossal (to muscles of the tongue): These fibers actually course anteriorly (see Figs. 21 and 23).

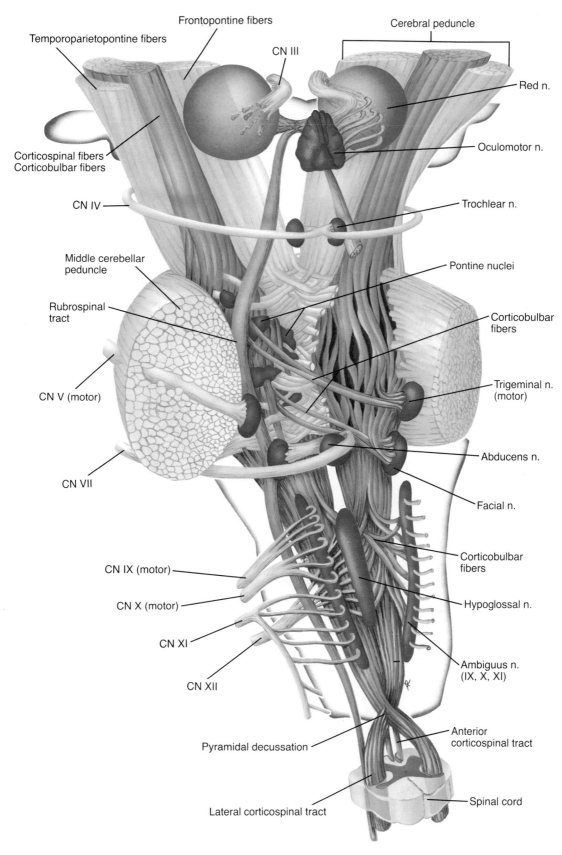

Temporoparietopontine fibers

Frontopontine fibers

CN III

Cerebral peduncle

Red n.

Oculomotor n.

Corticospinal fibers
Corticobulbar fibers

CN IV

Trochlear n.

Middle cerebellar
peduncle

Pontine nuclei

Rubrospinal
tract

Corticobulbar
fibers

CN V (motor)

Trigeminal n.
(motor)

Abducens n.

CN VII

Facial n.

Corticobulbar
fibers

CN IX (motor)

CN X (motor)

Hypoglossal n.

CN XI

Ambiguus n.
(IX, X, XI)

CN XII

Anterior
corticospinal tract

Pyramidal decussation

Spinal cord

Lateral corticospinal tract

FIGURE 48

119

FIGURE 49   # Reticular Formation and Pathways

The organization of the reticular formation has already been described (see Fig. 25). In this diagram, various nuclei that have significant (known) functional roles are depicted, as are the descending tracts emanating from some of these nuclei, again using the posterior perspective.

The reticular formation (RF) occupies the central portion or core area of the brain stem, from midbrain to medulla (Figs. 28 to 35). There are scattered nuclei in the midbrain region that seem to functionally belong to the reticular formation yet are not located within the core region. The periaqueductal gray and the locus ceruleus are also considered part of the reticular formation.

Topographically, the reticular formation can be described as being arranged in three longitudinal sets of neurons (see Fig. 25):

1   The *lateral group* consists of small neurons. These neurons receive the various inputs to the reticular formation. In this diagram, these neurons are shown receiving collaterals (or terminal branches) from the ascending anterolateral system, carrying pain and temperature (see Fig. 37). Similar information is received from the descending fibers of the trigeminal nerve. The reticular formation also receives visual and auditory information. The medial lemniscus, however, does not give off collaterals to the reticular formation.

2   The next group of neurons, situated more medially, is called the *central group*. These neurons are larger. Within this group are the well-known nucleus gigantocellularis of the medulla, and the pontine reticular nuclei, caudal and oral portions, located at the lower and upper pontine levels. Some of these cells project their axons upward or downward. The descending tracts that emanate from these nuclei are the medial and lateral reticulospinal pathways (see Figs. 44 and 45).

3   The *raphe nuclei* are a set of neurons that occupies the midline region of the brain stem. The best-known nucleus of this group is the *nucleus raphe magnus,* located in the upper part of the medulla (see Fig. 50).

The cerebral cortex sends fibers to the reticular formation nuclei, forming part of the so-called corticobulbar fibers. Nuclei that give off the pathways to the spinal cord form part of an indirect motor system—the corticoreticulospinal pathways. These pathways are known to have an important role in the voluntary control of the muscles of the spine (axial musculature) and of the large joints (proximal joints of the shoulder and hip). In addition, this system is known to play an extremely important role in the control of muscle tone. Lesions of the cortical input to the reticular formation in particular have a significant impact on muscle tone (discussed with Fig. 45). In humans, the end result is a state of increased muscle tone (spasticity), accompanied by an increase in the responsiveness of the deep tendon reflexes (hyperreflexia).

The periaqueductal gray of the midbrain is also often included with the reticular formation. It also receives input (illustrated but not labeled) from the ascending sensory systems conveying pain and temperature, the anterolateral and trigeminal. As shown in Figure 50, some of the neurons of the periaqueductal gray and the nucleus raphe magnus of the medulla are part of a descending pathway to the spinal cord concerned with pain control.

The *locus ceruleus* projects its noradrenergic fibers to virtually every part of the CNS, including all cortical areas, subcortical structures, the brain stem and cerebellum, and the spinal cord. Although the functional and electrophysiologic role of this pathway is still not clear, the locus ceruleus has been implicated in a wide variety of CNS activities.

The *serotonergic raphe nuclei* also project to all parts of the CNS. Again, the functional role of this system is not clear. Recent studies indicate that serotonin is important in sleep regulation and plays a significant role in emotional equilibrium.

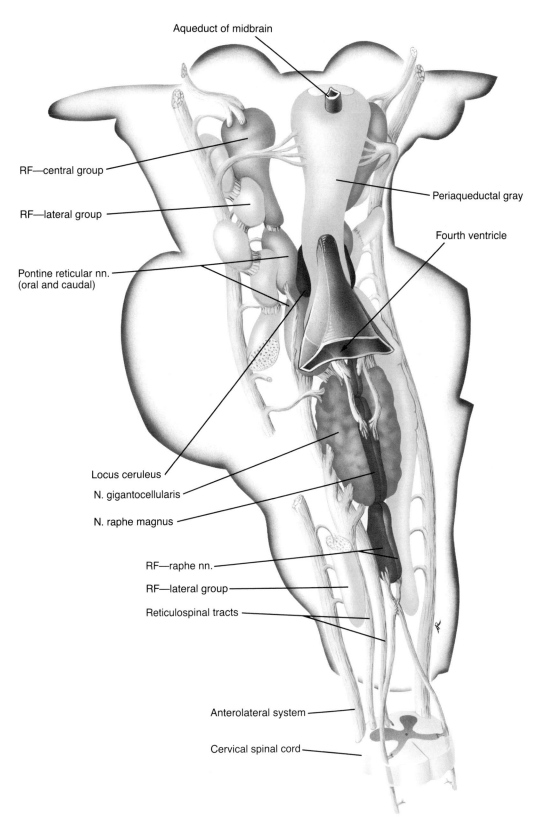

Aqueduct of midbrain

RF—central group

RF—lateral group

Pontine reticular nn.
(oral and caudal)

Periaqueductal gray

Fourth ventricle

Locus ceruleus

N. gigantocellularis

N. raphe magnus

RF—raphe nn.

RF—lateral group

Reticulospinal tracts

Anterolateral system

Cervical spinal cord

FIGURE 49

FIGURE 50   # Descending Pain System

Substantial evidence suggests that the transmission of pain from the periphery can be influenced by nuclei located in the brain stem. The areas that have been found to exert the major influence include the periaqueductal gray of the midbrain and the midline serotonergic nucleus of the medulla, the nucleus raphe magnus. The system apparently functions in the following way.

The neurons of the periaqueductal gray can be activated in a number of ways. Physiologically, it is known that many ascending fibers from the anterolateral system (and trigeminal system) activate neurons in this area (see Fig. 49). These are either collaterals of ascending pain fibers or direct endings of these fibers in the midbrain. This area is also known to be rich in opiate receptors, and it seems that neurons of this region can be activated by circulating endorphins. Experimentally, one can activate these neurons by direct stimulation or by a local injection of morphine. In addition, descending cortical fibers may also be available to activate these neurons.

The axons of some of the neurons of the periaqueductal gray descend and terminate in one of the raphe nuclei in the medulla. The particular nucleus is called *nucleus raphe magnus*. This nucleus is one of the serotonin-containing raphe system of nuclei (see Fig. 25).

From here, there is a descending, crossed pathway that is located in the dorsolateral funiculus of the spinal cord (shown but not labeled in Fig. 49). The serotonergic fibers terminate in the *substantia gelatinosa* of the spinal cord (see Fig. 64), a nuclear area of the dorsal horn of the spinal cord. The axons are thought to terminate on small interneurons that contain enkephalin.

It is postulated that these enkephalin-containing spinal neurons inhibit the transmission of the pain afferents in the spinal cord. This is the physiologic basis for the gate theory of pain. This theory also proposes that these same interneurons can be activated by stimulation of other sensory afferents, particularly those conveying information from the mechanoreceptors; these are anatomically large, well-myelinated peripheral nerve fibers.

The same mechanism is thought to be operative in the descending nucleus of the trigeminal nerve, the lower portion of which is responsible for pain (and temperature) transmission from the face. This nucleus is in fact continuous with the substantia gelatinosa.

Chronic pain is a particularly tragic state of being for many people. It is also often a difficult condition to treat. Some of the current treatments for chronic pain are based on the structures and neurotransmitters being discussed here. The gate theory underlies the use of transcutaneous stimulation, one of the current therapies offered for the relief of chronic pain. More controversial and certainly less certain (from the point of view of the physiologic basis) is the use of acupuncture in the treatment of pain.

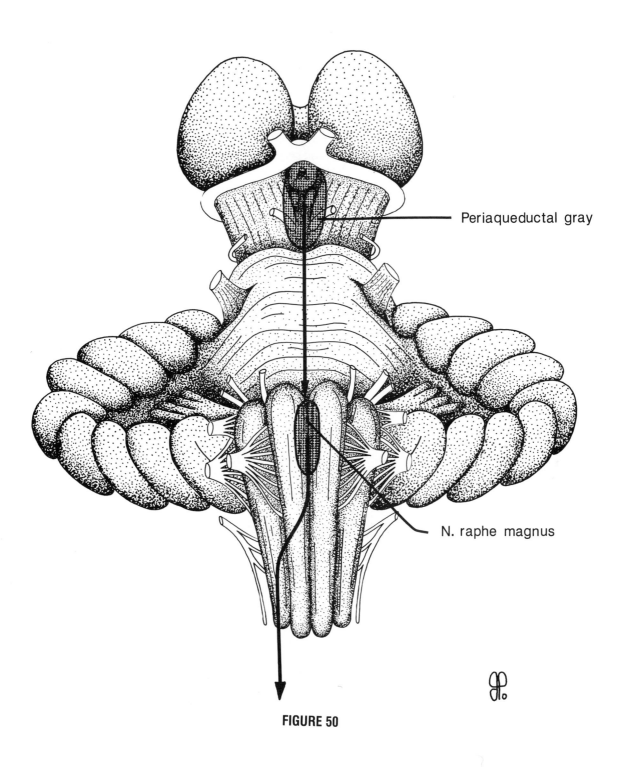

Periaqueductal gray

N. raphe magnus

FIGURE 50

FIGURE 51 # Medial Longitudinal Fasciculus

The MLF (medial longitudinal fasciculus) is a tract within the brain stem and upper spinal cord that links the visual world and vestibular events with the movements of the eyes and the neck, in addition to linking up the nuclei that are responsible for eye movements. The tract runs from the midbrain level to the upper thoracic level of the spinal cord. It has a rather constant location near the midline, dorsally, just anterior to the cerebral aqueduct and the fourth ventricle (see brain stem cross sections in Figs. 28 to 35).

Each of the component parts of the system can be considered separately:

Vestibular fibers: The four vestibular nuclei (see Fig. 24) receive much of their input from the *semicircular canals.* The lateral vestibular nucleus gives rise to the lateral vestibulospinal tract (see Figs. 43 and 65). Descending fibers originate in the medial vestibular nucleus and become part of the MLF; this can be called the *medial vestibulospinal tract.* There are also ascending fibers that come from the medial and superior vestibular nuclei that also are carried in the MLF. Therefore, the MLF carries both ascending and descending vestibular fibers.

Visuomotor fibers: Various nuclei are concerned with the movements of the eyes.

1 The three cranial nerve nuclei concerned with eye movements (III, IV, and VI) are located at different levels of the brain stem (see Fig. 23). If one considers lateral gaze, a movement of the eyes to the side (in the horizontal plane), this requires the coordination of the lateral rectus muscle (abducens nucleus) of one side and the medial rectus of the other side (oculomotor nucleus). These fibers for coordinating the eye movements are carried in the MLF.

2 There is thought to be a gaze center within the pontine reticular formation for saccadic eye movements, which are extremely rapid (ballistic) movements of both eyes yoked together, usually in the horizontal plane. These fibers likely course in the MLF.

Vision-related fibers: Visual information is received by various brain stem nuclei.

1 The *superior colliculus* is a nucleus for the coordination of vision-related reflexes, including eye movements and turning of the neck. It receives input from the spinal cord (spinotectal tract) and the visual association cortical areas, areas 18 and 19 (see Fig. 56A). The descending fibers from the superior colliculus, called the *tectospinal tract,* are closely associated with the MLF and can be considered part of this system (although they are discussed separately in most books). As shown in the upper inset, these fibers cross in the midbrain. (Note that the superior colliculus of only one side is shown so as not to obscure the crossing fiber systems at that level.)

2 A small nucleus in the periaqueductal gray region of the upper midbrain—the *interstitial nucleus* (of Cajal)—is also involved in the coordination of eye and neck movements. This nucleus receives input from various sources and contributes fibers to the MLF. Some prefer to call this the *interstitiospinal tract.*

The lower inset shows the MLF in the ventral funiculus of the spinal cord, at the cervical level (see Fig. 65). The three components of the tract are identified—those coming from the medial vestibular nucleus, the fibers from the interstitial nucleus, and the tectospinal tract. These fibers are mingled together in the MLF.

In summary, the MLF is a complex fiber bundle necessary for the proper functioning of the visual apparatus. The MLF interconnects the three cranial nerve nuclei responsible for movements of the eyes with the motor cells controlling the movements of the head and neck. It allows the visual movements to be influenced by vestibular, visual, and other information, and carries fibers (upward and downward) that coordinate eye movements with the turning of the neck.

The diagram also shows the *posterior commissure.* This small commissure carries fibers connecting the superior colliculi. In addition, it carries the important fibers for the consensual pupillary light reflex (discussed with the midbrain in Part B-II). The role of the commissural nuclei is not known.

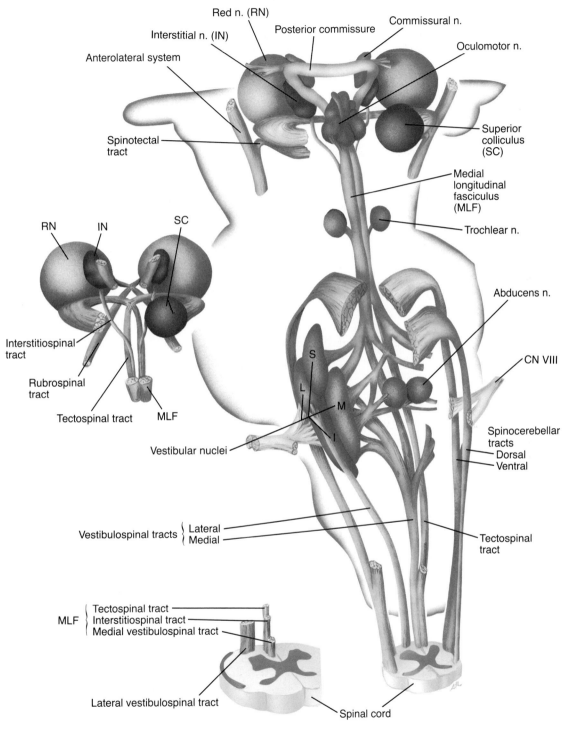

Red n. (RN)
Posterior commissure
Commissural n.
Interstitial n. (IN)
Oculomotor n.
Anterolateral system
Spinotectal tract
Superior colliculus (SC)
Medial longitudinal fasciculus (MLF)
Trochlear n.

RN   IN   SC

Interstitiospinal tract
Rubrospinal tract
Tectospinal tract   MLF

Abducens n.

CN VIII

S
L   M
I

Vestibular nuclei

Spinocerebellar tracts
Dorsal
Ventral

Vestibulospinal tracts { Lateral
Medial

Tectospinal tract

MLF { Tectospinal tract
Interstitiospinal tract
Medial vestibulospinal tract

Lateral vestibulospinal tract

Spinal cord

FIGURE 51

125

The Thalamus (Figures 52–57)

FIGURE 52

Thalamus: Orientation

The *diencephalon* is composed of the *thalamus* and *hypothalamus*. Translated as "between brain," the diencephalon is situated between the brain stem and the cerebrum. As shown in the photograph in Figure 22 and also diagrammatically in Figure 59, the diencephalon sits atop the brain stem. What has happened during the development of the human brain is an enormous growth in the cerebral hemispheres, which has virtually hidden or buried the diencephalon (somewhat like a weeping willow tree) so that it can no longer be visualized from the outside except from the inferior view (see hypothalamus in Fig. 4).

In this section of the *Atlas,* we consider the thalamus, which makes up the bulk of the diencephalon. The hypothalamus and other nuclear areas such as the habenula are discussed with the limbic system in Section G. The pineal (visible in Figure 22), which is sometimes considered a part of the diencephalon, will not be discussed. The area between the thalamus and midbrain, called the *subthalamic nucleus,* is involved with the circuitry of the basal ganglia and substantia nigra and is discussed with those structures (see Fig. 15).

As shown in the diagram, the diencephalon is situated within the brain below the level of the body of the lateral ventricles (and also below the level of the corpus callosum). In fact, the thalamus forms the "floor" of this part of the ventricle (see Figs. 19 and 55). In a horizontal section of the hemispheres, the two thalami are located at the same level as the lentiform nucleus (see Fig. 18); on each side, the thalamus forms one of the boundaries of the posterior limb of the internal capsule. Between the two thalami is the third ventricle (see Figs. 18 and 22). Some of these relationships can also be seen in a coronal section through the brain (see Fig. 19).

The thalamus is strongly linked with the cerebral cortex, even during development. This feature becomes clearer in one of the principles of thalamic function—that any thalamic nucleus that projects to the cerebral cortex also receives input from that area. These are called *reciprocal connections*. This principle does not apply, however, to all of the nuclei (as will be discussed with Fig. 53).

The various thalamic nuclei have different functions, which will be discussed in more detail with Figure 53. All the sensory systems have a synaptic relay in the thalamus before the information is sent on to the cerebral cortex, with the exception of the olfactory sense. Likewise, two subsystems of the motor system, the basal ganglia and the cerebellum, send their information to the cortex after a synaptic relay in the thalamus. In addition, the limbic system has circuits that involve the thalamus. Other thalamic nuclei are related to association areas of the cerebral cortex. Parts of the thalamus play an important role in the maintenance and regulation of the state of consciousness, alertness, and possibly attention.

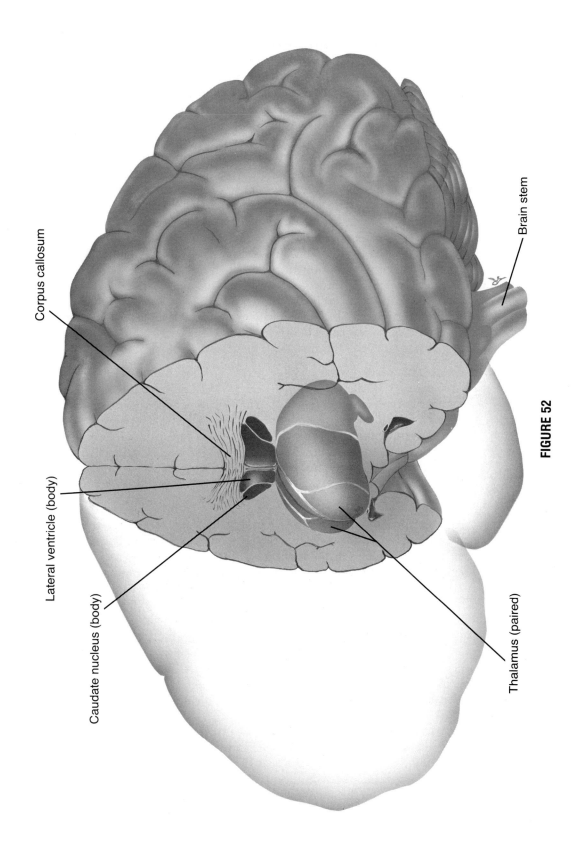

Corpus callosum

Lateral ventricle (body)

Caudate nucleus (body)

Thalamus (paired)

Brain stem

FIGURE 52

FIGURE 53 # Thalamus: Nuclei

As noted, the thalamus is composed of different nuclei that are part of different systems. There are two ways of dividing up the nuclei of the thalamus–(1) functionally. The thalamus has three different types of nuclei. Nuclei that relay sensory and motor information to specific sensory and motor areas of the cerebral cortex are called *specific relay nuclei*. Nuclei that are connected to broad areas of the cerebral cortex (known as the *association areas*) are called *association nuclei*. Nuclei that have other or multiple connections are classified as *nonspecific nuclei*. This functional group of nuclei does not have reciprocal connections with the cortex like the other nuclei. Some of these nonspecific nuclei form part of the ascending reticular activating system, which is involved in the regulation of our state of consciousness and arousal (discussed with Fig. 25). (2) Topographically. The thalamus is subdivided by bands of white matter into a number of component parts. The main white matter band that runs within the thalamus is called the *internal medullary lamina* and is shaped like the letter Y (see Figs. 52 and 80). It divides the thalamus into a lateral mass, a medial mass, and an anterior group of nuclei.

The basic subdivision of the thalamus into nuclear groups combines both the topographic and functional nomenclatures. For example, the specific relay nuclei are located in the lateral nuclear mass, and it is reasonable to include with these the medial and lateral geniculate bodies. The major nucleus of the medial mass is the *dorsomedial nucleus*. The nuclei located within the internal (medullary) lamina are functionally nonspecific and are often referred to as the *intralaminar nuclei*. The *reticular nucleus,* which lies on the outside of the thalamus, is also part of this functional system. The nuclei are organized as follows:

Specific relay nuclei
- ventral anterior (motor)
- ventral lateral (motor)
- ventral posterolateral (somatosensory)
- ventral posteromedial (trigeminal)
- medial geniculate (body) nucleus (auditory)
- lateral geniculate (body) nucleus (vision)

Association nuclei
- dorsomedial nucleus (prefrontal)
- anterior nucleus (limbic)
- pulvinar (visual)
- lateral dorsal (parietal)

Nonspecific nuclei
- intralaminar
- centromedian
- reticular

For schematic purposes, a presentation of the thalamic nuclei shown in a number of textbooks is quite usable. In reality, however, sections taken at different planes through the thalamus show different nuclei of varying size in a continuously changing configuration. In this diagram, the thalamus is shown at three different planes of section.

In the main diagram, the thalamus is "opened" in its middle to show some of the nuclei as well as the internal medullary lamina with its nuclei. Two other cuts have been made, one more anteriorly and the other posteriorly, showing the configuration of the different nuclei. The anterior cut includes the mammillary nucleus of the hypothalamus and the mammillothalamic tract that goes to the anterior nucleus of the thalamus; this is an association nucleus (actually a group of nuclei) that belongs to the limbic system and is discussed in Section G (see Fig. 79). In the posterior cut, the section goes through the lateral geniculate nucleus and shows that it is a laminated nucleus (see Fig. 56B); the medial geniculate nucleus and the pulvinar are also seen.

These diagrams show the relationship of the thalamus to adjacent structures. Above the thalamus is the body of the lateral ventricle, with the choroid plexus intervening. At the lateral edge of the ventricle is found the body of the caudate nucleus and the stria terminalis (see Fig. 76). Near the midline is the fornix, just below the corpus callosum (see Fig. 19). Lateral to the thalamus is the internal capsule; the posterior limb is seen in the anterior cut (see Figs. 17 and 18), with remnants of the lentiform nucleus and the so-called inferior limb (which is actually the auditory radiation [see Fig. 55]) in the posterior cut.

Both cuts include also the temporal lobe, with the inferior horn of the lateral ventricle, and the tail of the caudate nucleus in its upper aspect. Protruding into the ventricle is the hippocampus proper (see Figs. 76 and 77); the dentate gyrus is also present but not labeled.

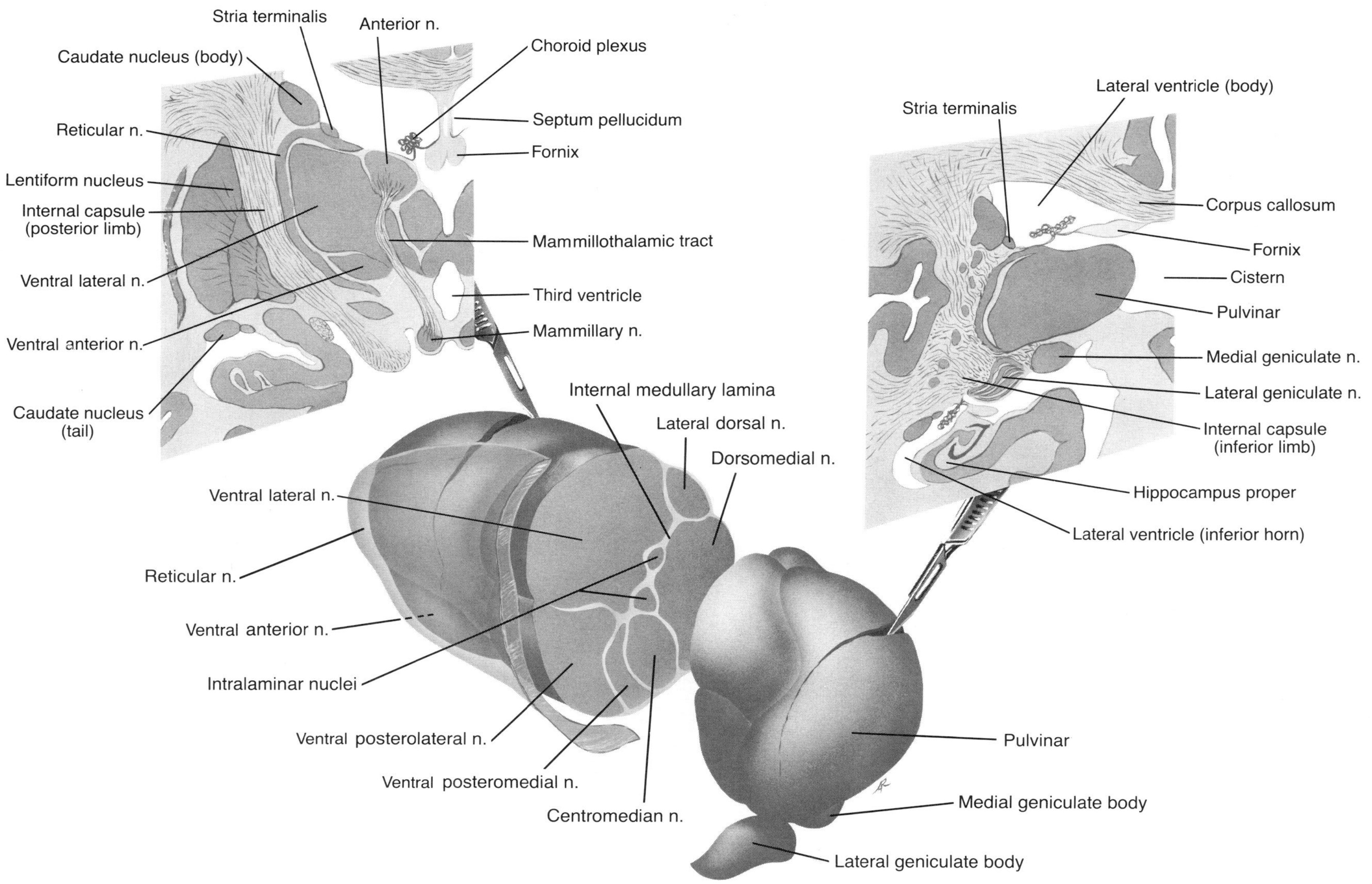

Lateral ventricle (body)
Corpus callosum
Fornix
Cistern
Pulvinar
Medial geniculate n.
Lateral geniculate n.
Internal capsule (inferior limb)
Hippocampus proper
Lateral ventricle (inferior horn)

Stria terminalis

Pulvinar
Medial geniculate body
Lateral geniculate body

Choroid plexus
Septum pellucidum
Fornix
Mammillothalamic tract
Third ventricle
Mammillary n.

Internal medullary lamina
Lateral dorsal n.
Dorsomedial n.

Anterior n.

Stria terminalis

Caudate nucleus (body)
Reticular n.
Lentiform nucleus
Internal capsule (posterior limb)
Ventral lateral n.
Ventral anterior n.
Caudate nucleus (tail)

Centromedian n.

Ventral lateral n.
Reticular n.
Ventral anterior n.
Intralaminar nuclei
Ventral posterolateral n.
Ventral posteromedial n.

FIGURE 53

131

FIGURE 54

Somatosensory and Trigeminal Systems

The brain stem pathway that carries discriminative touch sensation and information about joint position (as well as vibration) from the body is the *medial lemniscus* (see Fig. 36). The equivalent pathway for the face comes from the principal nucleus of the trigeminal nerve, which is located at the pontine level (see Figs. 24, 31, and 38). Most of this trigeminal system is crossed (TTc); there are also ascending trigeminal fibers that come from midline portions of the face that remain ipsilateral (TTi). The two come together forming the *trigeminal lemniscus.*

By the level of the midbrain, all of these sensory pathways, including the anterolateral system carrying pain and temperature sensation from the body (see Fig. 37), as well as the equivalent fibers (crossed) from the descending tract of V (see Fig. 47), merge together. This is shown in a series of cuts (in the lower portion of the diagram) through the midbrain region. At the level of the lower midbrain, these pathways are located near the surface, dorsal to the substantia nigra; as they ascend, they are found deeper within the midbrain, dorsal to the red nucleus (shown in cross section in Figs. 28 and 29).

The two pathways carrying the modalities of fine touch, position sense, and vibration terminate in different parts of a specific relay nucleus of the thalamus:

- medial lemniscus (from the body) in the ventral posterolateral nucleus
- trigeminal pathways (from the face) in the ventral posteromedial nucleus

Sensory modality and topographic information is retained in these nuclei. There is some physiologic processing of the sensory information, and some type of sensory "perception" occurs at the thalamic level. Precise localization and two-point discrimination are cortical functions.

After the synaptic relay, the pathways continue as the (superior) thalamocortical radiation through the posterior limb of the internal capsule and then into the white matter of the hemispheres. The somatosensory information is distributed to the cortex along the postcentral gyrus (see the small diagrams of the brain). The information from the face and hand is topographically situated on the dorsolateral aspect of the hemispheres (see Fig. 2). The information from the lower limb is localized along the continuation of this gyrus on the medial aspect of the hemispheres (see Fig. 7). Further elaboration of the sensory information occurs in the parietal association areas adjacent to the postcentral gyrus (the superior parietal lobule, known as areas 5 and 7).

The pathways carrying pain and temperature sensation from the body and the face terminate only partially in the specific relay nuclei. The smaller slower-conducting fibers terminate for the most part in the intralaminar nuclei. These terminations may well be involved with the emotional correlates that accompany many sensory experiences (e.g., pleasant or unpleasant).

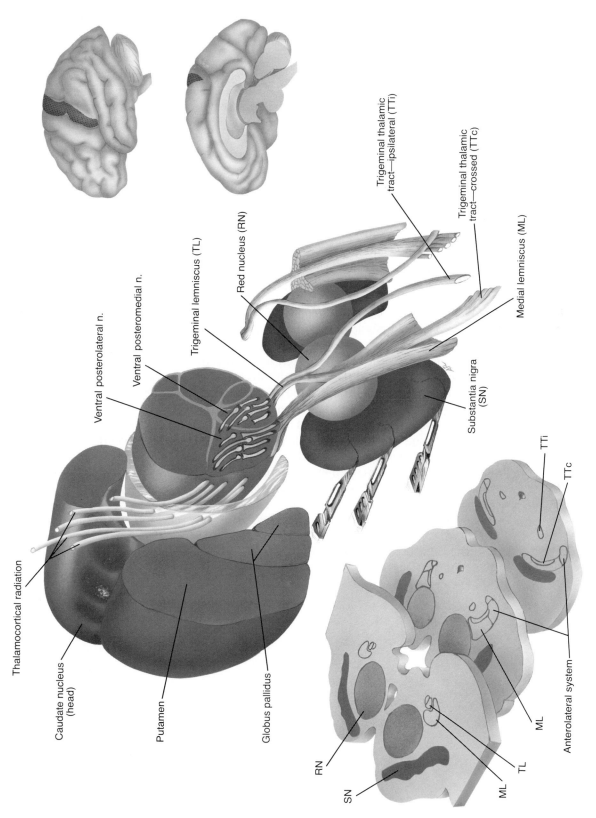

Trigeminal thalamic tract–ipsilateral (TTi)

Trigeminal thalamic tract–crossed (TTc)

Medial lemniscus (ML)

Red nucleus (RN)

Trigeminal lemniscus (TL)

Ventral posteromedial n.

Ventral posterolateral n.

Thalamocortical radiation

Caudate nucleus (head)

Putamen

Globus pallidus

Substantia nigra (SN)

RN

SN

ML

TL

ML

Anterolateral system

TTi

TTc

FIGURE 54

133

FIGURE 55   # Auditory System

Auditory information is carried via the *lateral lemniscus* to the *inferior colliculus* (see Figs. 39 and 47) after several synaptic relays. There is another synapse in this nucleus, making the auditory pathway overall somewhat different and more complex than the medial lemniscal and visual pathways. The inferior colliculi are connected to one another by a small commissure (not labeled).

The auditory information is next projected to a specific relay nucleus of the thalamus, the *medial geniculate body (nucleus)*. The tract that connects the two, the *brachium of the inferior colliculus,* can be seen on the dorsal aspect of the midbrain (see Fig. 22, not labeled; see Fig. 46); this is shown diagrammatically here.

From here, the auditory pathway continues to the cortex. This projection courses beneath the lentiform nucleus of the basal ganglia (see Part A-II). It is called the *sublenticular pathway,* the *inferior limb of the internal capsule,* or simply the *auditory radiation.* The cortical areas involved with receiving this information are the *transverse gyri of Heschl,* situated on the superior temporal gyrus. The location of these gyri is shown in the inset as the primary auditory areas (also seen in a photographic view in Fig. 3).

Sound frequency, known as *tonotopic organization,* is maintained all along the auditory pathway, starting in the cochlea. This can be depicted as a musical scale with high and low pitches. The auditory system localizes the direction of a sound in the superior olivary complex (see Fig. 32) by analyzing the difference in the timing that information reaches each ear and by the difference in sound intensity that reaches each ear. The loudness of a sound would be represented physiologically by the number of receptors stimulated and by the frequency of impulses, as in other sensory modalities.

The medial geniculate nucleus is likely involved with some analysis and integration of the auditory information. More exact analysis occurs in the cortex. Further elaboration of auditory information is carried out in the adjacent cortical areas. On the dominant side for language, these cortical areas overlap Wernicke's area (see Fig. 2).

The view of the brain shown in this illustration includes the body of the lateral ventricle (cut) and adjoining structures. The thalamus is seen to form the floor of the ventricle; the body of the caudate nucleus lies above the thalamus and on the lateral aspect of the ventricle. Just adjacent to it is the stria terminalis (not labeled). The temporal lobe structures are also shown, including the inferior horn of the lateral ventricle, the hippocampus proper and adjoining structures (as in Fig. 53), the stria terminalis, and the tail of the caudate nucleus.

This diagram also includes the lateral geniculate body (nucleus), which subserves the visual system, and its projection, the optic radiation, which commences in the same general area (discussed with the next illustration).

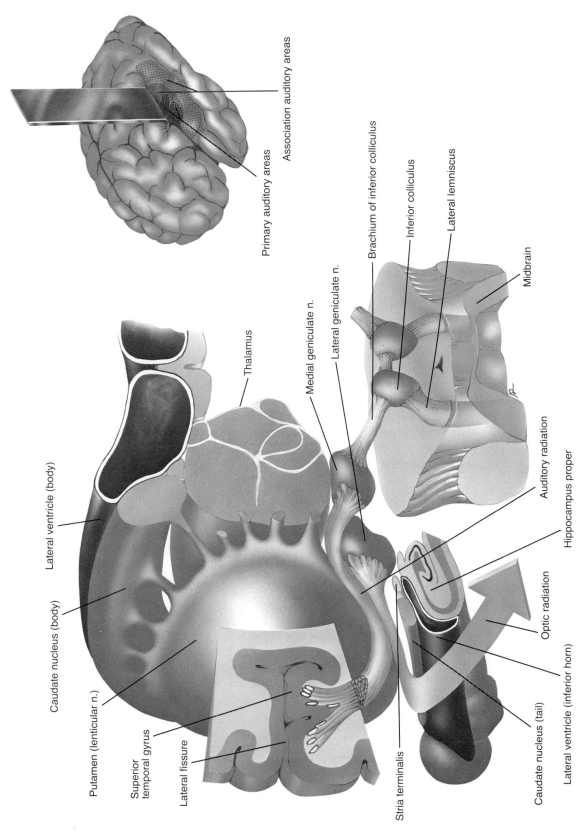

Association auditory areas

Primary auditory areas

Brachium of inferior colliculus

Inferior colliculus

Lateral lemniscus

Midbrain

Thalamus

Medial geniculate n.

Lateral geniculate n.

Lateral ventricle (body)

Caudate nucleus (body)

Putamen (lenticular n.)

Superior temporal gyrus

Lateral fissure

Stria terminalis

Auditory radiation

Hippocampus proper

Optic radiation

Caudate nucleus (tail)

Lateral ventricle (inferior horn)

FIGURE 55

FIGURE 56A   # Visual System—A

In the opinion of many, modern humans have become most dependent on vision. It is through our visual sense that we gain access to information (the written word), the world of images (e.g., photographs, television), and the complex urban landscape.

Visual processing begins in the retina with the *photoreceptors.* The *bipolar neurons,* the first neurons in the chain, are functionally equivalent to cells in the dorsal root ganglion of the somatosensory system, or the bipolar neurons of the spiral ganglion for hearing. The next neuron in a sensory system has axons that cross the midline and project to the thalamus (e.g., the nuclei gracilis and cuneatus). In the visual system, these are the *ganglion cells* of the retina, whose axons form the *optic nerve,* cross (only some cross) in the *optic chiasm,* continue in the *optic tract,* and terminate in the *lateral geniculate nucleus* (see Fig. 53). In fact, this whole pathway from ganglion cells to geniculate, although it is known as CN II, in reality is a pathway of the central nervous system, with the oligodendrocyte being the myelin-forming cell. In mammals, the optic nerve is not known to regenerate following injury.

The fibers from the retina synapse in different layers of the lateral geniculate nucleus (discussed with the next diagram). After the processing that occurs here, fibers project to the *visual cortex.* The projection is unusual (discussed in more detail in Fig. 56B), with some of the fibers sweeping forward alongside the inferior horn of the lateral ventricle in the temporal lobe while others project directly posteriorly. The sweep of fibers in the temporal horn is called the *temporal loop (Meyer's loop).* The whole *geniculocalcarine projection,* from thalamus to cortex, eventually becomes situated behind the lenticular nucleus and is called the *retrolenticular projection* of the internal capsule, or simply the *visual* or *optic radiation.*

The visual information goes to area 17 (shown in black in the insets), the primary visual area. This is located in part at the occipital pole and mainly on the medial surface of the hemispheres along the banks of the calcarine fissure (see Fig. 7). The cortex along the calcarine fissure represents mostly the peripheral areas of the retina and is supplied by the posterior cerebral artery (from the vertebrobasilar system). The macular area of the retina is represented mostly at the occipital pole and is usually supplied by the middle cerebral artery (from the internal carotid system). The adjacent cortical areas of the occipital lobe, areas 18 and 19, are association areas for vision.

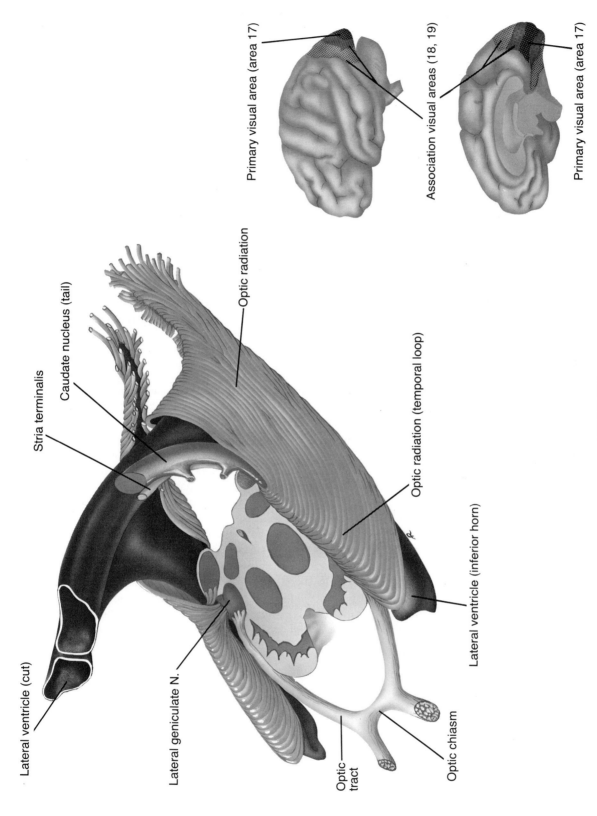

Lateral ventricle (cut)

Stria terminalis

Caudate nucleus (tail)

Lateral geniculate N.

Optic tract

Optic chiasm

Optic radiation

Optic radiation (temporal loop)

Lateral ventricle (inferior horn)

Primary visual area (area 17)

Association visual areas (18, 19)

Primary visual area (area 17)

FIGURE 56A

137

FIGURE 56B   # Visual System—B

There is only a partial crossing of fibers in the optic chiasm—that is, only those axons from the medial half of the retina cross in the chiasm. Functionally, this means that the visual field from one side is represented in the optic tract (and geniculate and cortex) on the opposite side.

Most fibers of the optic tract project to the *lateral geniculate nucleus*. This nucleus has a six-layered structure (see also Fig. 53), similar to the lamination seen in the cortex; the presence of lamination in a noncortical structure is unusual. Each of the eyes projects to specific layers of this nucleus, in fact, to three of the layers. The projection is said to occur "in register," so that corresponding points from the two eyes project to adjacent parts of the lamina. This is another indication that the information about the visual field is retained in the visual pathway.

The *geniculocalcarine (optic) projection,* which eventually lies alongside the occipital horn of the lateral ventricle, is arranged in the following manner:

- The fibers that represent the lower retinal field (upper visual field) sweep forward into the temporal lobe (temporal loop; see Fig. 56A) and terminate in the cortex of the lower bank of the calcarine fissure. Destruction of these fibers on one side results in a loss of vision in the upper visual field of the opposite side—specifically, the upper quadrant of both eyes.
- Those fibers representing the upper retinal field (lower visual field) project posteriorly without this unusual looping, pass deep within the parietal lobe, and terminate in the cortex of the upper bank of the calcarine fissure. Destruction of these fibers on one side results in the loss of the lower visual field of the opposite side—specifically, the lower quadrant of both eyes.

The illustration shows some fibers from the optic tract that project to the *superior colliculus* (bypassing the lateral geniculate) via the brachium of the superior colliculus. This nucleus serves as an important center for visual reflex behavior, particularly that involving eye movements. Fibers leave this nucleus and connect with the nuclei of the extraocular and neck muscles via the medial longitudinal fasciculus (see Fig. 51). There is also a projection to the spinal cord via the tectospinal tract, which is found incorporated with the medial longitudinal fasciculus throughout the brain stem and the upper spinal cord.

Other fibers are illustrated emerging from the *pulvinar,* the vision-related association nucleus of the thalamus. These are carried in the optic radiation and go to areas 18 and 19, the visual association areas of the cortex; they are shown in the previous diagram, alongside area 17 (on both the dorsolateral and medial surfaces of the brain).

Other fibers from the optic tract (not shown) project to the *pretectal area,* which is situated anterior (and superior) to the superior colliculus. The reflex adjustment of the diameter of the pupil—the pupillary light reflex—is coordinated in the pretectal nucleus (discussed with the midbrain in Part B-II). Some other fibers terminate in the *suprachiasmatic nucleus* of the hypothalamus (located above the optic chiasm), which is involved in the control of diurnal (day–night) rhythms.

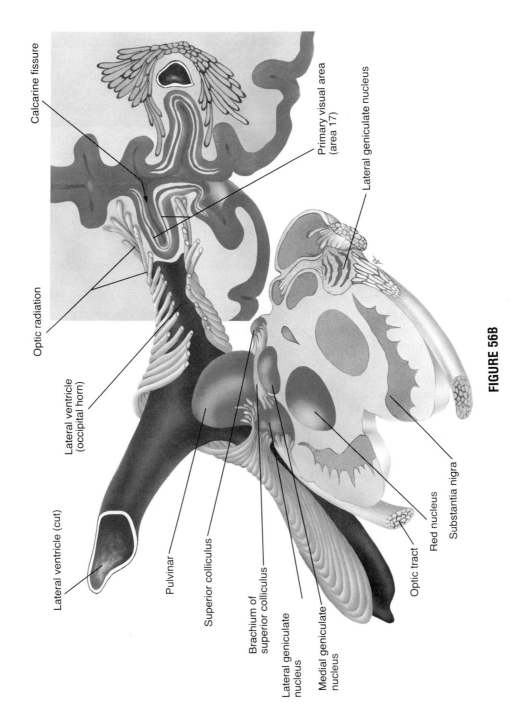

Calcarine fissure

Optic radiation

Lateral ventricle
(occipital horn)

Lateral ventricle (cut)

Pulvinar

Superior colliculus

Brachium of
superior colliculus

Lateral geniculate
nucleus

Medial geniculate
nucleus

Optic tract

Red nucleus

Substantia nigra

Primary visual area
(area 17)

Lateral geniculate nucleus

FIGURE 56B

FIGURE 57   # Motor Circuits

The specific relay nuclei of the thalamus that are linked with the motor system are the *ventral lateral* and the *ventral anterior nuclei*. These project to different cortical areas involved in motor control. One of the intralaminar nuclei, the *centromedian nucleus,* is also linked with the motor system.

The major outflow from the basal ganglia is from the medial segment of the globus pallidus. Two slightly different pathways project to the thalamus—*pallidothalamic fibers*—one passing around and the other passing through the fibers of the internal capsule (represented on the diagram by large stippled arrows). These merge and end in the ventral anterior and ventral lateral nuclei of the thalamus. (The ventral anterior nucleus is not seen on this diagram.) These nuclei also receive input from the substantia nigra, pars reticulata. The cortical projection is to the *premotor* and *supplementary motor* areas (see inset diagrams).

The functional contribution of the basal ganglia to the motor system has been discussed previously (with Fig. 12). The precise role that these thalamic nuclei play in this pathway is still not clear. Clinically, a lesion in the thalamic region that interrupts this pathway or destroys part of these nuclei has been shown to alleviate some of the symptoms of Parkinson's disease. The theory is that the surgical removal of impulses restores the balance between the various inputs to the cortical areas involved in motor control.

The other subsystem of the motor system, the cerebellum, also projects to the cortex via the thalamus. The dentate nucleus, the largest of the deep cerebellar nuclei and the one that receives input from the neocerebellum, projects its fibers via the superior cerebellar peduncle (see Figs. 47 and 63). Some of the fibers may terminate in the red nucleus. The major projection—the *cerebellothalamic fibers*—is to the ventral lateral nucleus, but to a different portion of it than it receives from the basal ganglia. From here, the fibers project to the motor areas of the cerebral cortex—namely, the *motor* area of the precentral gyrus and the *premotor* area (areas 4 and 6).

Functionally, the neocerebellum seems to be involved in motor planning (discussed in the introduction to Section E). Again, it is not easy to understand what role the thalamus plays in integrating this information, prior to the projection to the cerebral cortex.

The areas of the cerebral cortex that receive input from these two subsystems of the motor system are shown diagrammatically, on both the dorsolateral and medial surfaces of the hemispheres. As noted, the cortical areas and the thalamic nuclei are reciprocally interconnected.

The pathway involving the *centromedian nucleus* is rather distinct. The afferents come from the medial segment of the globus pallidus. Efferents from the centromedian nucleus go to the caudate-putamen, hence forming a feedback loop to the basal ganglia (discussed with Fig. 15).

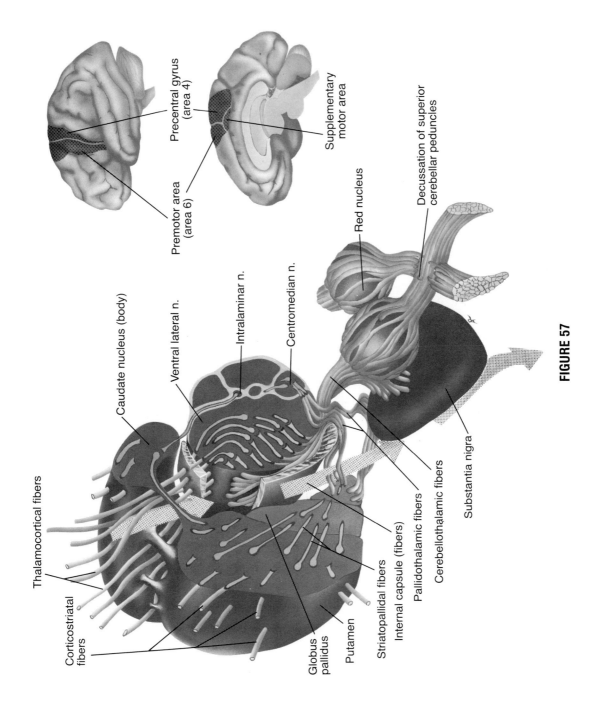

Precentral gyrus (area 4)

Premotor area (area 6)

Supplementary motor area

Decussation of superior cerebellar peduncles

Red nucleus

Caudate nucleus (body)

Ventral lateral n.

Intralaminar n.

Centromedian n.

Thalamocortical fibers

Corticostriatal fibers

Globus pallidus

Putamen

Striatopallidal fibers

Internal capsule (fibers)

Pallidothalamic fibers

Cerebellothalamic fibers

Substantia nigra

FIGURE 57

141

· ·

The Cerebellum (Figures 58–63)

INTRODUCTION

The cerebellum is involved with motor control and is part of the motor system, influencing posture, gait, and voluntary movements. Its function is to facilitate the performance of movements by coordinating the action of the various participating muscle groups. This is often spoken of simply as "smoothing out" motor acts. Although it is rather difficult to explain what the cerebellum does in motor control, damage to the cerebellum leads to dramatic alterations in ordinary movements. Lesions of the cerebellum result in decomposition of activity, or fractionation of movement, so that the action is no longer smooth and coordinated. Certain cerebellar lesions also produce a tremor seen when performing voluntary acts, better known as an *intention tremor*.

The cerebellum is organized with cortical tissue on the outside, the *cerebellar cortex*. The cortex consists of three layers, and all parts appear to be structurally alike. The most important cell of the cortex is the *Purkinje neuron,* whose massive dendritic system "processes" the cerebellar inputs. The Purkinje cell axon leaves the cortex and projects to the cell groups deep within the cerebellum, the *intracerebellar* (deep cerebellar) *nuclei.* Increased firing of the Purkinje neuron inhibits the ongoing activity of these deep cerebellar nuclei, whereas decreased Purkinje cell firing results in a decrease in the inhibitory effect on the deep cerebellar cells—that is, this results in the increased firing of the deep cerebellar neurons.

The cerebellum receives information from many parts of the nervous system, including the spinal cord, the vestibular system, the brain stem, and the cerebral cortex. Projecting to the cerebellar cortex, these afferents are excitatory and influence the ongoing activity of the neurons in the intracerebellar nuclei. The Purkinje neuron activity is altered by the various inputs, an alteration reflected as an increase or decrease in the inhibitory effect of the Purkinje cells on the deep cerebellar nuclei. Axons from the deep nuclei neurons project from the cerebellum to many areas of the central nervous system. In this way, the cerebellum exerts its influence on motor performance. The various connections are carried in the three cerebellar peduncles—the superior, middle, and inferior. Each attaches the cerebellum to a part of the brain stem.

Anatomically, the cortex of the cerebellum is divided into areas and lobes (which have Latin names). Essentially, there is the central portion, called the *vermis,* and the remainder, which constitutes the *lateral lobes.* Other lobes (e.g., the *anterior lobe*) can be subdivided according to the major fissures found, but many of the other named areas do not have (as yet) any functional correlation. There are four deep cerebellar nuclei—the *fastigial* nucleus (most medial), the *globose* and *emboliform* nuclei (intermediate), and the lateral or *dentate* nucleus.

More important is the division of the cerebellum on the basis of its functional units, of which it has three—the vestibulocerebellum, the spinocerebellum, and the neocerebellum. Each of these includes a cortical component and a part of the deep cerebellar nuclei.

Note: The following information should be reviewed after the student has studied the cerebellum with the aid of the illustrations in this section.

Vestibulocerebellum

This is thought to be the oldest part of the cerebellum (the archicerebellum). Afferents come from the vestibular system and the vestibular nuclei. These enter the cerebellum through the inferior cerebellar peduncle. The regions of the cerebellum concerned with this information include the *nodulus* (part of the vermis) and the *flocculus* (i.e., the *flocculonodular* lobe). After cortical processing, the fibers project to the *fastigial* nucleus; from here, axons leave the cerebellum and go to the brain stem. Lesions of the vestibulocerebellum produce a disturbance of equilibrium (balance) and gait, and may give rise to nystagmus (rhythmical oscillations of the eyes).

Spinocerebellum

Afferents are derived from the muscle spindles and the joints. The major part of this input enters the cerebellum through the inferior cerebellar peduncle, and the remainder enters alongside the superior cerebellar peduncle (see Fig. 47). The information is processed in the spinal part of the cerebellum, which consists of several parts—most of the anterior lobe, most parts of the vermis, and a strip of cerebellum lying adjacent to the vermis, called the *intermediate zone*. The axons from this region project to the fastigial nucleus as well as to two other intracerebellar nuclei, the *globose* and *emboliform* (together called the *intermediate nucleus*). Their fibers project to the brain stem as well. An important function of this part of the cerebellum is that of a *comparator* comparing ongoing activity with motor commands related to the particular movement. Lesions of the spinocerebellum affect muscle tone and may also have an effect on posture and gait.

Cerebrocerebellum (Neocerebellum)

This functional portion includes most of the *lateral lobes* of the cerebellum. From an evolutionary perspective, it is the most recent area to develop. The input to this part of the cerebellum includes wide areas of the cerebral cortex, with a predominance coming from the motor areas. These are conveyed through descending corticopontine fibers that relay (synapse) in the pontine nuclei (see Fig. 31) and enter the cerebellum through the massive middle cerebellar peduncles. After cortical processing, the fibers project to the *dentate nucleus,* which sends its axons to certain nuclei of the thalamus (see Fig. 57). These thalamic nuclei project to the motor portions of the cerebral cortex, thus influencing motor control. Lesions of the neocerebellum result in the classic symptoms of the decomposition of voluntary movements (discussed with Fig. 63), as well as an intention tremor that occurs when attempting to perform voluntary actions. It is thought that the neocerebellum is also involved in motor planning.

FIGURE 58

Cerebellum: Lobes

The cerebellum is located in the skull beneath the tentorium cerebelli, in the posterior cranial fossa. It lies inferior to the occipital lobe of the hemispheres (see Fig. 2).

As seen in the photograph (see Fig. 4), the surface of the cerebellum is thrown into small folds, called *folia*. *Sulci* separate each of these, and some of the deeper sulci may be termed *fissures*. This allows the division of the cortex into a number of different lobes. The folia in these drawings are represented schematically.

The human cerebellum in situ has an upper, or superior, surface and a lower, or inferior, surface (see Figs. 21 and 22). The *horizontal fissure* is located at the margin between the two surfaces (see Fig. 22). The appearance of the cerebellum can also be described in the following way. There is a central portion known as the *vermis*. The lateral portions are called the *cerebellar hemispheres*. On the superior surface, the vermis is elevated; on the inferior surface, the vermis lies in a depression between the hemispheres. When the brain is sectioned in the sagittal plane, the various portions of the cerebellar vermis can be identified (see Fig. 7). The most anterior part of the vermis on the superior aspect is the *lingula*. The most anterior piece of the vermis on the inferior aspect is the *nodulus*. A strip of tissue adjacent to the vermis is called the *intermediate* (paravermal) *zone*.

One of the main fissures, the *primary fissure,* is found on the superior surface. The cerebellar tissue in front of it constitutes the *anterior lobe* of the cerebellum. As already noted, most of the anterior lobe is part of the functional *spinocerebellum*. Both the vermis area and the intermediate zones are indicated on this representational view of the cerebellum. The functional spinocerebellum includes most of the vermis, together with the intermediate zone (both of which continue into the anterior lobe).

With the exception of the vermis and the adjacent strip (the intermediate zone), the tissue behind the primary fissure composes the *neocerebellum*. This continues onto the inferior surface of the cerebellum, until the dorsal aspect of the medulla is reached.

The *flocculus* is a small lobule of the cerebellum located on its inferior surface and oriented in a transverse direction, below the middle cerebellar peduncle (see Figs. 4 and 21). The flocculus is connected to the *nodulus,* the last piece of vermal tissue on the inferior surface of the cerebellum (see Fig. 7). Together they form the *flocculonodular lobe,* the functional *vestibulocerebellum.*

There is a convention of portraying the surface of the cerebellum as if it is found in a single plane. This is done in the following way. Using the lingula and the nodulus, the cerebellum is "opened up," placing the nodulus at the bottom of the diagram. The best analogy is to use a book, with the binding toward you. If you place the fingers of your right hand on the edge of the front cover (the lingula) and the fingers of your left hand on the edge of the back cover (the nodulus), you can (gently) open up the book so as to expose both the front and back covers. The front cover is the surface of the superior part of the cerebellum, and the back cover is the inferior surface. Both are now laid out in a single plane.

This same portrayal can be done with an isolated cerebellum and attached brain stem in the following way. The brain knife is introduced at the pontomedullary junction and directed toward the horizontal fissure. Before reaching the fissure, the superior and inferior surfaces are (gently) pulled apart, thereby making it possible to lay the cerebellum down on a flat surface, using the horizontal fissure as the "hinge" (equivalent to the binding of the book).

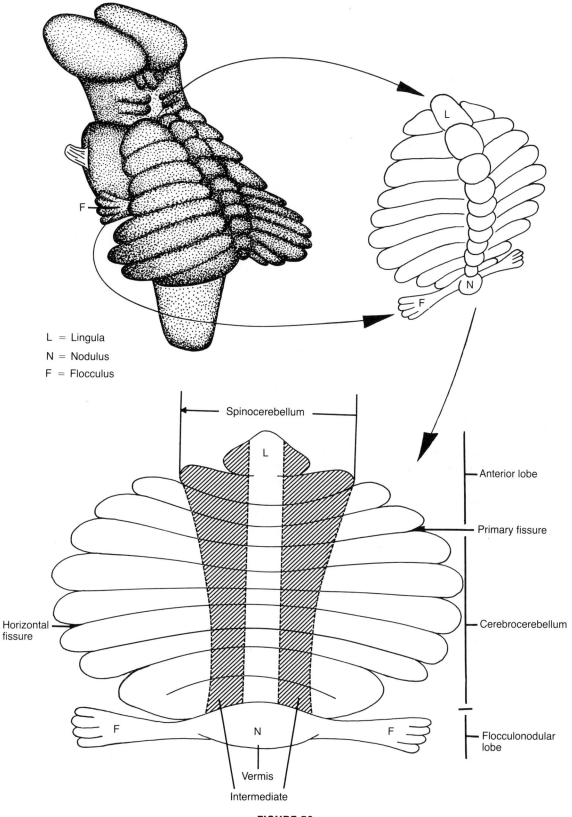

L = Lingula
N = Nodulus
F = Flocculus

Spinocerebellum

L

Anterior lobe

Primary fissure

Cerebrocerebellum

Horizontal
fissure

F   N   F

Flocculonodular
lobe

Vermis

Intermediate

FIGURE 58

147

FIGURE 59   # Cerebellum: Ventral View

The ventral view of the brain stem also includes the inferior aspect of the cerebellum. This is the same view as that in the photograph of the isolated brain stem and cerebellum (see Fig. 21).

The *flocculus* is shown as a separate piece of cerebellar tissue, oriented in a transverse direction. It seems to attach to the cerebellum at the cerebellopontine angle, with CN VIII just superior to it.

Attaching the pons to the cerebellum, on this view, is the large *middle cerebellar peduncle*. All portions of the cortex project to the pons as the corticopontine fibers (see Figs. 40 and 48). These synapse in the pontine nuclei and are relayed, after crossing, to the cerebellum, by means of this peduncle. This massive projection of cerebral cortex to the cerebellum is thought to provide information mainly to the neocerebellum; the neocerebellum processes this incoming data, and it is postulated that this is the part of the cerebellum involved in motor planning. The output from this part of the cerebellum is from the dentate nucleus, which projects through the superior cerebellar peduncle to the thalamus (see Figs. 47 and 63). The motor areas of the cerebral cortex receive this cerebellar information (discussed with Fig. 57).

The cerebellar lobule adjacent to the medulla is known as the *cerebellar tonsil* (see Fig. 21). The tonsils are found just inside the foramen magnum of the skull. Should there be an increase in the mass of tissue occupying the posterior cranial fossa (e.g., tumor or hemorrhage), the cerebellum would be pushed downward. This may force the cerebellar tonsils into the foramen magnum, thereby compressing the medulla. The compression, if severe, can lead to a compromising of function of the vital centers located in the medulla (discussed with Fig. 25). This is a life-threatening situation that can cause cardiac or respiratory arrest. The complete syndrome is known as *tonsillar herniation*.

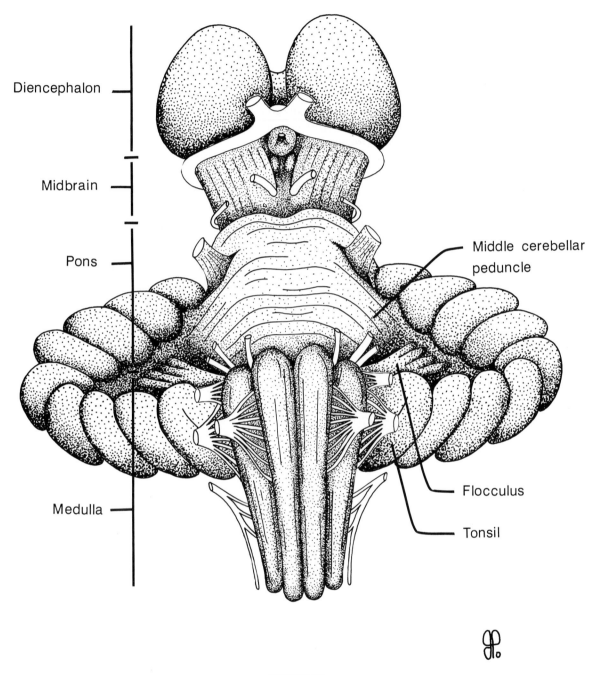

Diencephalon

Midbrain

Pons

Medulla

Middle cerebellar
peduncle

Flocculus

Tonsil

FIGURE 59

149

FIGURE 60

Intracerebellar Nuclei: Ventral View

The position of the deep cerebellar (intracerebellar) nuclei, which are located within the cerebellum, is indicated. Their location is superimposed on the ventral view of the cerebellum. (The intracerebellar nuclei are shown from a posterior perspective in Figure 62.)

The nuclei are arranged in the following manner:

1 The *fastigial* (*medial*) nucleus is located next to the midline.

2 The *globose* and *emboliform* nuclei are slightly more lateral; these often are grouped together and called the *intermediate* or *interposed nucleus*.

3 The *dentate nucleus*, with its irregular margin, is most lateral. This nucleus is sometimes called the *lateral nucleus* and is by far the largest.

The nuclei are located within the cerebellum at the level of the junction of the medulla and the pons. Therefore, the cross sections shown at this level (see Fig. 32) include these deep cerebellar nuclei. Usually, only the dentate nucleus can be identified in the real sections. The same holds true in gross anatomy laboratories for sections of the whole brain stem and cerebellum at this level.

The projection of the fastigial nuclei is almost completely to the brain stem. Some of this runs adjacent to the inferior cerebellar peduncle (discussed with Fig. 61). The interposed nuclei project to the brain stem and to the red nucleus; the projection to the red nucleus is via the superior cerebellar peduncle (see Fig. 57).

The dentate nucleus projection is the largest, and these fibers exit the cerebellum through the superior cerebellar peduncle (see Figs. 47 and 63). Their projection is to the thalamus (ventral lateral nucleus) and from there to the motor areas of the cerebral cortex (see Fig. 57).

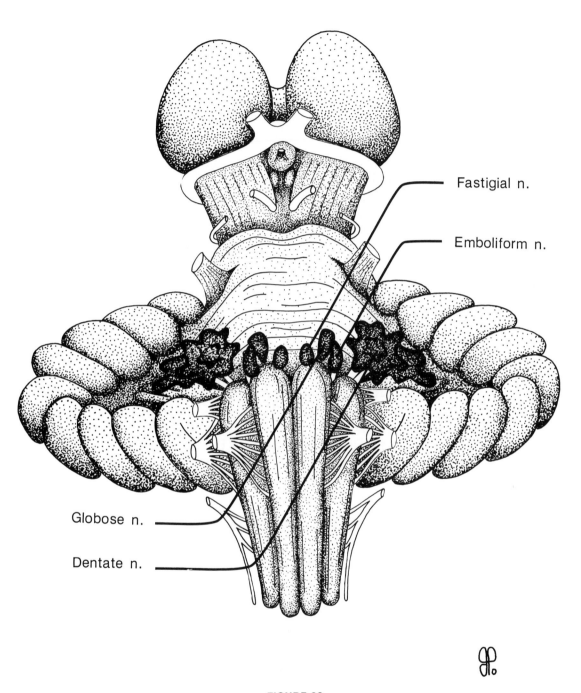

Fastigial n.

Emboliform n.

Globose n.

Dentate n.

FIGURE 60

FIGURE 61   # Cerebellum: Inferior Cerebellar Peduncle

The inferior cerebellar peduncle attaches the medulla to the cerebellum. It lies behind the inferior olivary nucleus and can sometimes be seen on the ventral view of the brain stem (as in Fig. 21).

This peduncle conveys a number of fiber systems to the cerebellum. These are shown schematically in this diagram of the ventral view of the brain stem and cerebellum. They include the following:

- The *posterior (dorsal) spinocerebellar pathway* is conveying proprioceptive information from most of the body. This is one of the major tracts of the inferior peduncle. These fibers, carrying information from the muscle spindles as well as from cutaneous sources, relay in the dorsal nucleus of Clarke in the spinal cord (see Fig. 64). They ascend ipsilaterally in a tract found at the edge of the spinal cord (see Figs. 51 and 65). These fibers are distributed to the spinocerebellar areas of the cerebellum.
- The homologous tract for the upper limb is the *cuneocerebellar tract*. It also enters the cerebellum by means of the inferior peduncle, conveying proprioceptive information from the upper extremity to the spinocerebellum. These fibers relay in the accessory (external) cuneate nucleus in the lower medulla (see Fig. 35). This pathway is not shown in the diagram.
- The *olivocerebellar tract* is also carried in this peduncle. The fibers originate from the inferior olivary nucleus (see Figs. 21 and 35), cross in the medulla, and are distributed to all parts of the cerebellum. These axons have been shown to be the climbing fibers to the main dendritic branches of the Purkinje neuron.
- Other cerebellar afferents from other nuclei of the brain stem, including the reticular formation, are conveyed to the cerebellum via this peduncle.

Efferent fibers from the fastigial nuclei to the brain stem exit from the cerebellum in a bundle found adjacent to the inferior cerebellar peduncle. The rather awkward name of this bundle of fibers, the *juxtarestiform body,* is derived from an older terminology: the inferior cerebellar peduncle used to be called the *restiform body*. It is unlikely that a student will be exposed to this terminology in a clinical setting, except perhaps in neuroradiology.

The *ventral spinocerebellar pathway* enters the cerebellum adjacent to the superior cerebellar peduncle (see Fig. 51; discussed with Fig. 63). As noted, the middle cerebellar peduncle conveys the massive input from the pontine nuclei (see Fig. 59).

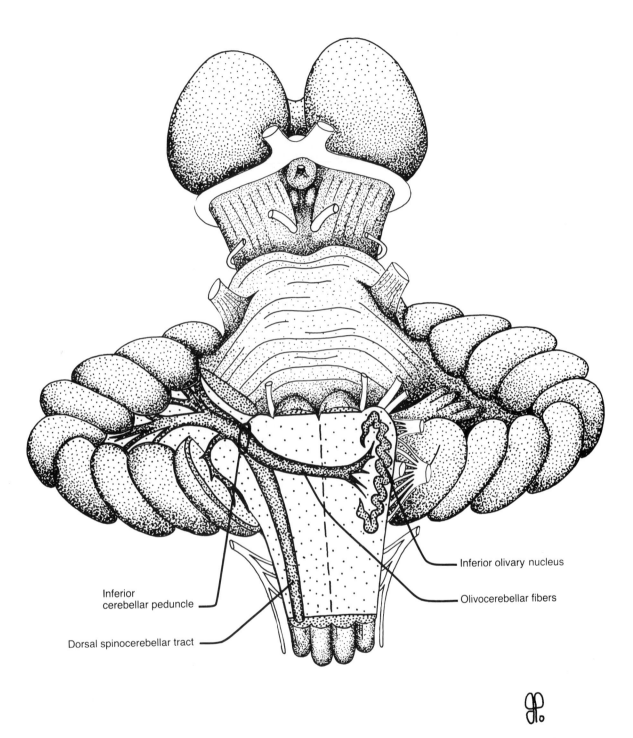

Inferior
cerebellar peduncle

Dorsal spinocerebellar tract

Inferior olivary nucleus

Olivocerebellar fibers

FIGURE 61

FIGURE 62

Cerebellum: Dorsal View

This view of the cerebellum is similar to that in the photograph of this view of the brain (see Fig. 22). It is a dorsal view of the diencephalon and midbrain. The third ventricle is situated between the two diencephala, with the interconnecting massa intermedia. The pineal gland is seen attached to the posterior aspect of the thalamus. Below are the superior and inferior colliculi.

The superior surface of the cerebellum can be seen. The vermis includes a group of midline folia that are elevated. In front of the primary fissure is the anterior lobe, part of the spinocerebellum. The remainder of this aspect of the cerebellum includes the intermediate area adjacent to the midline vermis, which is part of the spinocerebellum (see Fig. 58), and the lateral portions, which belong to the neocerebellum.

The location of the horizontal fissure is also indicated, separating the superior surface from the inferior one. The perspective of this diagram is such as to include several folia belonging to the inferior surface of the cerebellum.

The intracerebellar nuclei are depicted within the cerebellum, as if they could be seen from the outside. (This is similar to the view presented from the ventral perspective in Figure 60.) Their location within the cerebellum can be correlated with the projection they receive from the cerebellar cortex (please refer to Fig. 58 and review the introduction to this section).

1 The fastigial nuclei are centrally located and receive fibers from the vermis.
2 The emboliform and globose nuclei are the intermediate nucleus, and they receive fibers from the intermediate zone of the cerebellum, including most of the anterior lobe.
3 The dentate nucleus is most lateral and receives input from the lateral lobes of the cerebellum, which is almost exclusively the neocerebellum.

(The output of these nuclei was discussed with Figure 60 and in the introduction.)

The cerebellar cortex projects fibers directly to the lateral vestibular nucleus. As would be anticipated, these are inhibitory. The lateral vestibular nucleus (see Fig. 32) could therefore, in some sense, be considered one of the intracerebellar nuclei. This nucleus also receives input from the vestibular system and then projects to the spinal cord (see Fig. 43).

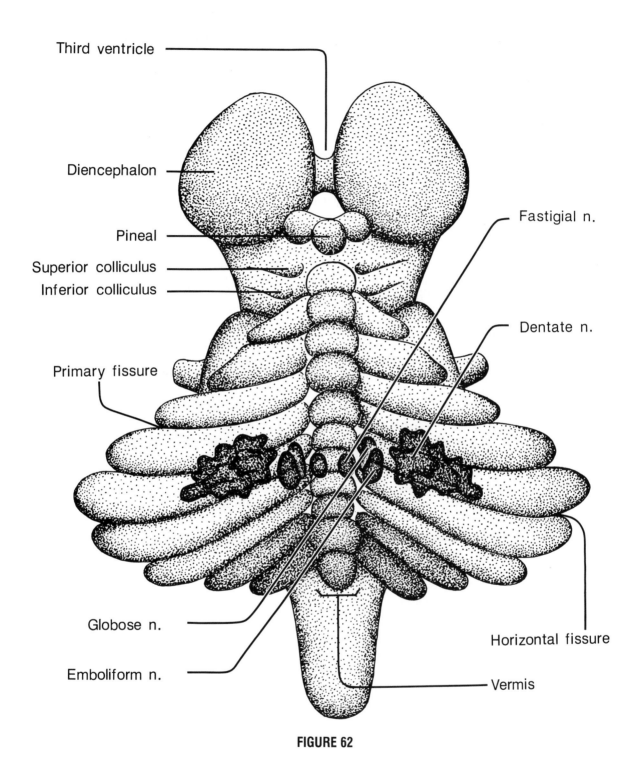

Third ventricle

Diencephalon

Pineal

Superior colliculus

Inferior colliculus

Primary fissure

Globose n.

Emboliform n.

Fastigial n.

Dentate n.

Horizontal fissure

Vermis

FIGURE 62

FIGURE 63

Cerebellum: Superior Cerebellar Peduncle

The superior cerebellar peduncle is the major outflow tract of the cerebellum. Associated with it are some of the cerebellar afferents conveyed in the ventral spinocerebellar pathway. This peduncle connects the cerebellum with the midbrain.

One group of cerebellar afferents, those carried in the *ventral (anterior) spinocerebellar* tract, enters the cerebellum by means of the superior cerebellar peduncle. These fibers cross in the spinal cord, ascend (see Figs. 51 and 65), enter the cerebellum, and cross again, thus terminating on the side from which they originated. (The dorsal spinocerebellar fibers terminate ipsilaterally as well.)

The outflow fibers originate mainly from the dentate nucleus, with some from the intermediate nucleus (not shown). The axons start laterally and converge toward the midline, coursing through the dorsal aspect of the pons (see Figs. 30 and 31). In this part of their course, they are located in the roof of the upper half of the fourth ventricle. Some fibers that form a bridge between the superior cerebellar peduncles in this area are named the *superior medullary velum* (discussed with Fig. 7; see also Fig. 46). From this dorsal perspective, it is possible to visualize the superior cerebellar peduncles in the gross brain specimen; these peduncles and the superior medullary velum can be seen by displacing the cerebellar tissue of the anterior lobe (below the inferior colliculi).

In the lower midbrain (see Fig. 29), there is a complete *decussation* of fibers. Some of the fibers terminate in the red nucleus of the midbrain, particularly those from the interposed nucleus. Most of the fibers, particularly those from the dentate nucleus, terminate in the *ventral lateral nucleus* of the thalamus (see Figs. 53 and 57). From here, they are relayed to the motor cortex, areas 4 and 6.

Therefore, the neocerebellum is linked to the cerebral cortex by a circuit that forms a loop. Fibers are relayed through the pons from the cerebral cortex to the cerebellum. The pontocerebellar fibers are crossed and go to the neocerebellum of the opposite side. After cortical processing, the neocerebellar fibers project to the dentate nucleus. The efferents project to the thalamus, after decussating in the lower midbrain. From the thalamus, fibers are relayed mainly to the motor areas of the cerebral cortex. Because of the two crossings, the messages are returned to the same side of the cerebral cortex from which the circuit began.

Lesions of the neocerebellum of one side cause motor deficits to occur on the same side of the body—that is, ipsilaterally. The explanation for this lies in the fact that the corticospinal tract is also a crossed pathway (see Figs. 41 and 48). For example, the errant messages from the left cerebellum that are delivered to the right cerebral cortex cause the symptoms to appear on the left side (i.e., ipsilaterally) from the point of view of the cerebellum.

The cerebellar symptoms associated with lesions of the neocerebellum (or the superior cerebellar peduncle) involve the range, direction, and amplitude of voluntary actions. Groups of muscles no longer function cooperatively in matters of timing and sequencing. This failure of muscular coordination is often called *cerebellar ataxia*. The specific symptoms include the following:

- Distances are improperly gauged when pointing, a symptom called *dysmetria* and that includes pastpointing.
- Rapid alternating movements are poorly performed, called *dysdiadochokinesia*.
- Complex movements are performed as a series of successive isolated movements, which is called a *decomposition of movement* (dyssynergia).
- Disturbances occur in the normally smooth production of words, resulting in slurred and explosive speech.
- A tremor is seen during voluntary movement, called an *intention tremor*. (This is in contrast to the parkinsonian tremor, which is present at rest and disappears during voluntary movement.)

In addition, cerebellar lesions in humans are often associated with hypotonia and sluggish deep tendon reflexes.

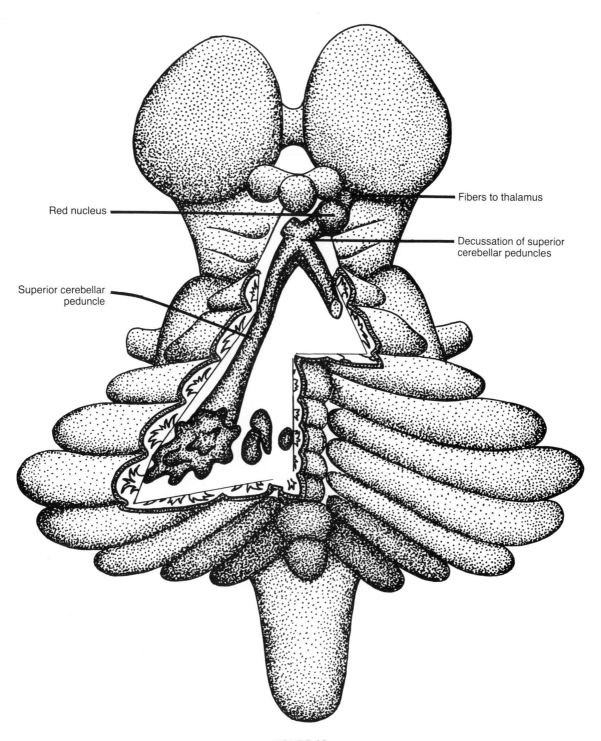

Red nucleus

Fibers to thalamus

Decussation of superior
cerebellar peduncles

Superior cerebellar
peduncle

FIGURE 63

The Spinal Cord (Figures 64–69)

INTRODUCTION

The spinal cord is an elongated mass of nervous tissue that, despite its relatively small size (compared with the rest of the brain), is essential for our normal function. On the motor side, the descending tracts "instruct" the motor neurons (the anterior horn cells), either directly or indirectly. This enables us to carry out normal movements, including walking and the so-called voluntary activities and the associated movements. On the sensory side, the information arriving from the skin, muscles, and viscera informs the central nervous system about what is occurring in the periphery.

Embryologically, the spinal cord commences as a tube of uniform size. In the segments that innervate the limbs (muscles and skin), all the neurons reach maturity. Massive cell death occurs in the intervening portions, however, because there is less peripheral tissue to be supplied. In adults, therefore, the spinal cord has two "enlargements"—the cervical for the upper limb and the lumbosacral for the lower limb. The spinal cord ends at the L2 vertebral level in adults, and at a lower level (L4) in young children. The *lumbar cistern* (with CSF) continues inferiorly, containing the dorsal and ventral roots (the *cauda equina*).

Anatomically, the spinal cord is divided into gray matter (with the neurons) and white matter (with the tracts). The gray matter is located in the interior and is surrounded by the white matter. It is said to be arranged in the shape of a butterfly. The ventral gray matter, called the *ventral horn,* is the motor portion of the spinal cord gray matter. The dorsal gray matter, called the *dorsal horn,* is the sensory portion. The area between the horns is often called the *intermediate gray* and has a variety of cell groups with some association-type functions.

The white matter surrounds the gray matter and is divided by it into three areas—the dorsal, lateral, and anterior areas. These zones are sometimes referred to as *funiculi* (single, *funiculus*). Various tracts are located in each of these three zones, some ascending and some descending.

Physiologically, the spinal cord is the basis of a number of reflexes, simple (e.g., myotatic or stretch) and complex (e.g., the withdrawal reflex from painful stimuli). Recent studies indicate that complex motor patterns are present in the spinal cord, such as stepping movements with alternating movements of the limbs, and that influences from higher centers provide the organization for these built-in patterns of activity. The integrity of the spinal cord is needed for normal bowel and bladder function.

Lesions of the human spinal cord are often devastating in their effects. They often occur as the result of diving accidents (into shallow water) or car accidents. If the spinal cord is completely transected (i.e., cut through), all the tracts are interrupted. As for the ascending pathways, this means that sensory information from the periphery is no longer available to the brain. On the motor side, all the motor commands cannot be transmitted to the anterior horn cells, the final common pathway for the motor system. The person therefore is completely cut off on the sensory side and loses all voluntary control below the level of the lesion. Bowel and bladder control are also lost.

In humans, the immediate effect of a spinal cord transection is a complete shut-down of spinal cord activity. This is referred to as *spinal shock*. Neurologically, there is a loss of muscle tone and an absence of deep tendon reflexes, although the *Babinski sign* (discussed with Fig. 41) is present. After a few weeks, intrinsic spinal reflexes appear, accompanied by a dramatic increase in muscle tone (spasticity) and hyperactive deep tendon reflexes (hyperreflexia). Thereafter, a number of abnormal or excessive reflex responses occur. Such patients require exceptional care by the nursing staff. The exact symptoms vary with each patient, depending on the level of the lesion and the amount of injury to the spinal cord.

Each segment of the spinal cord supplies an area of skin, called the *dermatome,* and a number of muscles, known as the *myotome*. Therefore, destruction of the gray matter leads to segmentally detectable changes, usually if a few adjacent segments of the cord are damaged. These deficits must be differentiated from damage to the exiting nerve roots.

Clinical examination of the patient can usually determine the level of a transection. A hemitransection (in which half the cord is damaged) is called *Brown-Séquard syndrome*. Since the blood supply to the spinal cord is tenuous, spinal cord damage can occur after a period of cardiovascular shock from a variety of causes. Various diseases can lead to a degeneration of specific tracts of the spinal cord, such as amyotrophic lateral sclerosis, in which there is a degeneration of the lateral corticospinal tract (due to loss of motor cells of the cerebral cortex), as well as death of the anterior horn cells. Finally, scattered lesions affecting any number of tracts and leading to a variety of symptoms can be seen in the demyelinating disease multiple sclerosis.

FIGURE 64

Spinal Cord Cross Section: Nuclei—C8 Level

The gray matter of the spinal cord contains a variety of cell groups, or nuclei. The various nuclei subserve different functions. Although it is rather hard to visualize, these groups are continuous longitudinally throughout the length of the spinal cord.

The dorsal region of the gray matter (the *dorsal horn*) is associated with the incoming dorsal root and is thus related to sensory functions. The *ventral horn* has the large anterior horn cells and is related to motor functions. The area in between is the *intermediate gray*.

The nuclei of the spinal cord gray matter have both names and numbers. The names are older and are descriptive. A newer numbering-system classifies these nuclei on a functional basis; these are known as the *Rexed laminae*. This cross section of the spinal cord shows the descriptive names on the left side and the Rexed laminae on the right.

Name	Lamina	Function
Posteromarginal nucleus	I	Sensory
Substantia gelatinosa	II	Sensory
Proper sensory nucleus	III, IV	Sensory
Intermediate gray	V, VI, VII	Association
Dorsal nucleus (of Clarke)	Part of VII	Relay to cerebellum (dorsal spinocerebellar tract)
Ventral horn	VIII	Motor (axial muscles)
Groups of motor neurons (in ventral horn)	IX	Limb musculature Medial = proximal Lateral = distal
Commissural neurons	X	Unknown

Note: Missing from these diagrams is a small canal, the central canal of the spinal cord (see Figs. 10A and 10B). Located in the center of the commissural gray matter, it represents the remnant of the neural tube and is filled with cerebrospinal fluid (CSF). The central canal of the spinal cord is probably partially obliterated in the adult, and is therefore not shown in these figures.

A pathologic enlargement of the central canal can occur, usually in the cervical region. This disease process involves the pain and temperature fibers, after they have synapsed in the dorsal horn and as they are crossing to form the anterolateral system (see Fig. 37). The clinical result is a loss of pain and temperature sensation in a segmental fashion, often affecting the hand. The disease is called *syringomyelia*.

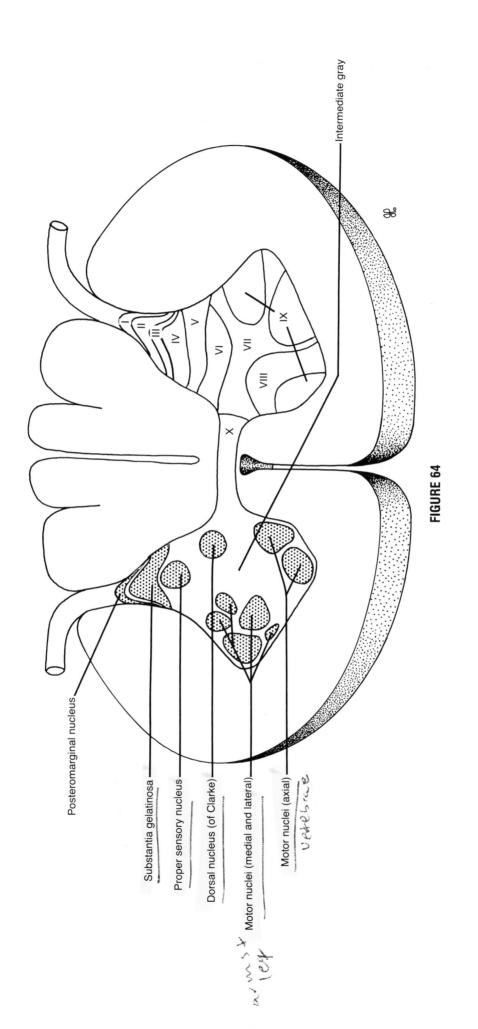

Intermediate gray

I
II
III
IV
V
VI
VII
VIII
IX
X

Posteromarginal nucleus

Substantia gelatinosa

Proper sensory nucleus

Dorsal nucleus (of Clarke)

Motor nuclei (medial and lateral)

Motor nuclei (axial)

vertebrae

arm st
leg

FIGURE 64

FIGURE 65

Spinal Cord Cross Section: Tracts—C8 Level

The major tracts of the spinal cord are shown on this diagram, the descending tracts on the left side and the ascending ones on the right. In fact, both sets are present on both sides.

Descending tracts
- Lateral corticospinal, from the cerebral cortex. These fibers cross in the lowermost medulla (see Figs. 40 and 48).
- Anterior (ventral) corticospinal, also from the cortex. These fibers do not cross in the pyramidal decussation (see Fig. 48).
- Rubrospinal, from the red nucleus. This tract crosses at the level of the midbrain (see Figs. 42, 48, and 51).
- Lateral vestibulospinal, from the lateral vestibular nucleus. This pathway remains ipsilateral (see Figs. 43 and 51).
- Lateral and medial reticulospinal tracts, from the medullary and pontine reticular formation, respectively (see Figs. 44, 45, and 49).
- Medial longitudinal fasciculus (MLF) which descends to the cervical spinal cord level (see Fig. 51).

Ascending tracts
- Dorsal column tracts, consisting at this level of both the fasciculus cuneatus and fasciculus gracilis (see Figs. 36 and 47).
- Anterolateral system, consisting of the anterior (ventral) spinothalamic and lateral spinothalamic tracts (see Figs. 37, 47, and 49).
- Spinocerebellar tracts, anterior (ventral) and posterior (dorsal) (see Fig. 51).

Special tract
- Dorsolateral fasciculus, better known as the *tract of Lissauer,* carries intersegmental information, particularly relating to pain afferents.

   Note to the student: The functional aspects of these tracts should be reviewed at this time.

Fasciculus gracilis

Fasciculus cuneatus

Posterior
spinocerebellar tract

Medial
longitudinal fasciculus

Anterior
spinocerebellar tract

Lateral
spinothalamic tract

Anterior
spinothalamic tract

Anterior
corticospinal tract

Dorsolateral fasciculus

Lateral
corticospinal tract

Rubrospinal tract

Pontine
reticulospinal tract

Medullary
reticulospinal tract

Vestibulospinal tract

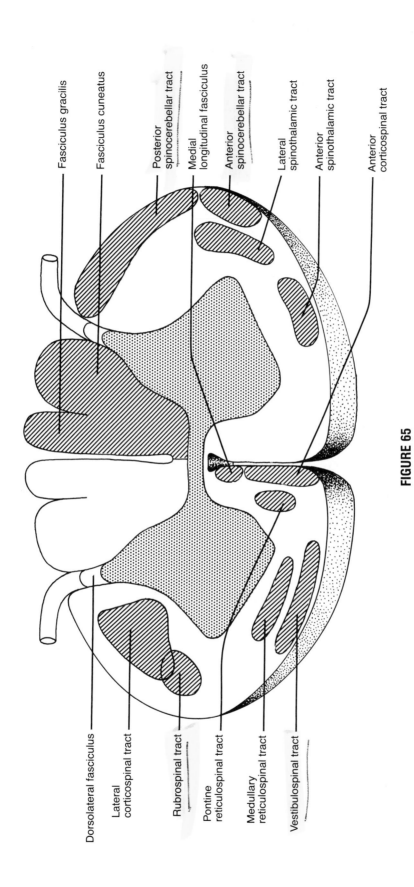

FIGURE 65

FIGURE 66

Cross Section of Spinal Cord: Cervical Level—C8

This is a section of the spinal cord through the cervical enlargement. The gray matter ventrally is very large because of the number of neurons involved in the innervation of the upper limb, particularly the muscles of the hand. The dorsal horn is likewise large, because of the amount of afferents coming from the skin of the fingers and hand.

The white matter is large in comparison with lower regions for the following reasons:

1   All the ascending tracts are present and are carrying information from the lower parts of the body as well as the upper limb.
2   The descending tracts are fully represented, since many of the fibers terminate in the cervical region of the spinal cord. Some of them do not descend to lower levels (e.g., MLF).

Note to the student: It is recommended that the student work out the clinical deficits that might be seen following a hemisection of the spinal cord at this level, on the right side.

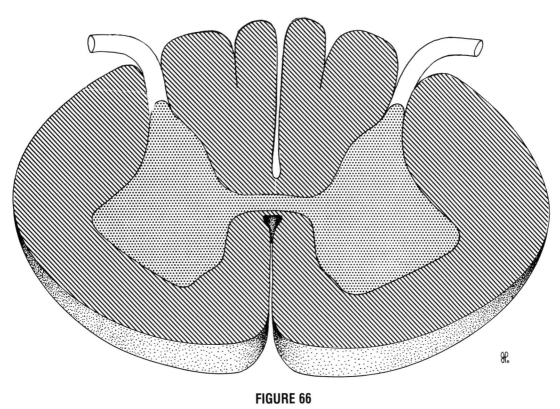

FIGURE 66

FIGURE 67   # Cross Section of Spinal Cord: Thoracic Level—T4

The thoracic region of the spinal cord presents an altered morphology because of the decrease in the amount of gray matter. As explained earlier, there are fewer muscles and less dense skin innervation in the thoracic region.

The gray matter has, in addition, a *lateral horn,* which represents the sympathetic neurons. This cell group, the *intermediolateral nucleus,* is the preganglionic sympathetic portion of the autonomic nervous system. The lateral horn is present throughout the thoracic region of the spinal cord and also the upper segments of the lumbar region.

The white matter of the thoracic region tapers slowly as it descends, because additional afferents are being added at higher levels and because descending tracts are terminating continuously.

The main blood supply to the spinal cord comes from two branches, one from each vertebral artery. These two small arteries join and form the *anterior spinal artery,* which descends in the midline, between the ventral funiculi. This artery receives supplementary branches from the aorta along its way, *radicular arteries,* which follow the nerve roots.

Clinically, the blood supply to the midthoracic region is marginally adequate. Therefore, any process that affects the systemic circulation (e.g., surgery, cardiovascular shock) may impair the blood supply here and lead to an infarction of the spinal cord.

Note to the student: The student is encouraged to work out the clinical symptoms that follow infarction of the complete spinal cord at this level.

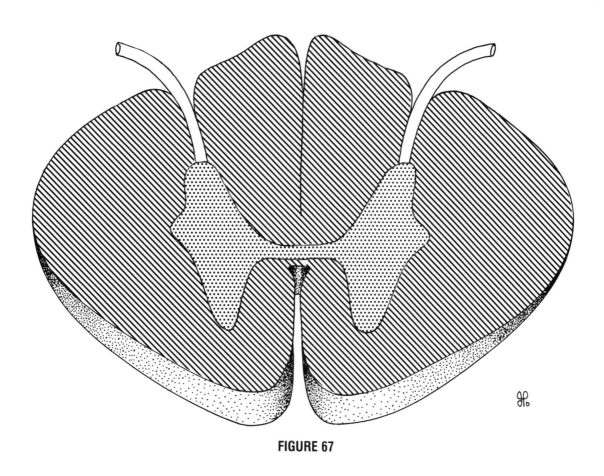

FIGURE 67

FIGURE 68 # Cross Section of Spinal Cord: Lumbar Level—L3

This cross section of the spinal cord is similar in appearance to the cervical section, because both are innervating the limbs. There is, however, proportionately less white matter at the lumbar level. The descending tracts are smaller because many of the fibers have terminated at higher levels. The ascending tracts are smaller because they are conveying information only from the lower regions of the body.

By this level of the spinal cord, the spinal cord segments do not match the vertebral level in adult humans. This is because the spinal cord usually ends, in fact, at the vertebral level L2. Below this level, the vertebral canal is filled with nerve roots, better known as the *cauda equina* (like a horse's tail). The CSF space in that region is the *lumbar cistern,* which is most commonly used for the sampling of CSF (i.e., a *lumbar puncture*).

The nerve roots exit the spinal cord at the appropriate intervertebral level. The roots to the lower extremity, those exiting between L4–L5 and L5–S1, are the ones most commonly involved in everyday back injuries that affect many adults. The student should be familiar with the signs and symptoms that accompany degenerative disk disease in the lumbar region.

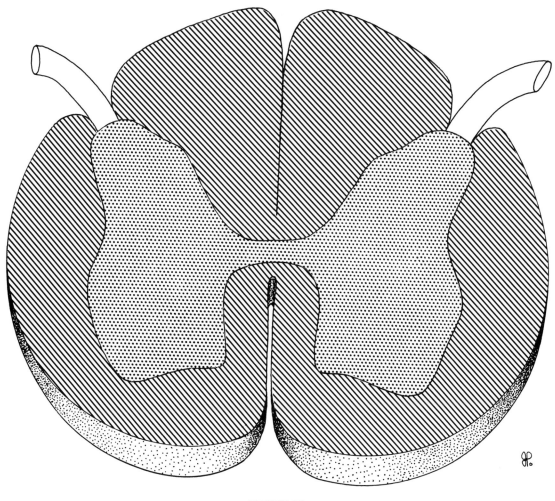

FIGURE 68

FIGURE 69

Cross Section of Spinal Cord: Sacral Level—S3

The sacral region of the spinal cord is the smallest and is therefore easy to recognize. The white matter is reduced in size. There is still a fair amount of gray matter because of the innervation of the pelvic musculature.

This region of the spinal cord also contains the *preganglionic parasympathetic* neurons of the autonomic nervous system innervating the pelvic viscera, including the bowel and the bladder. The conical termination of the spinal cord containing spinal segments S2 to S4 is called the *conus medullaris*. Injury to this region results in serious problems in the regulation of bowel and bladder functions.

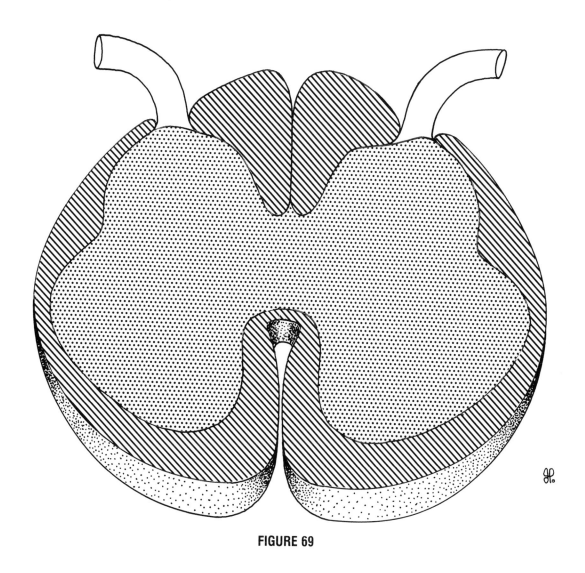

FIGURE 69

The Limbic System
(Figures 70–82B)

• •

INTRODUCTION

The *limbic system* is a term that is almost synonymous with the term *emotional brain*. All of us are aware of what we mean when we use the terms *emotions,* and *feelings,* yet they are somewhat difficult to define precisely. *Stedman's Medical Dictionary* defines *emotion* as "a strong feeling, aroused mental state, or intense state of drive or unrest directed toward a definite object and evidenced in both behavior and in psychologic changes." Thus, emotions involve:

> *Behavior:* The animal or human does something, that is, performs some type of motor activity, such as displaying anger, fighting, mating, and, in humans, smiling or laughing, or verbalizing. Both cortical and subcortical areas of the brain may be involved.

> *Physiologic changes:* These may include basic drives involving thirst, sexual behavior, and appetite. These are often manifested as changes involving the autonomic nervous system. The hypothalamus and pituitary gland are the structures underlying the hormonal responses.

> *Alterations in the mental state:* These can be understood as a change in the way we feel or react. Another way of describing these alterations is to introduce the idea of "emotional tone": with an increase in tone we may feel elated or tense; with a decrease, sad or lethargic. Humans are sometimes able to describe and verbalize their reactions or the way they feel. It is generally assumed that lower animals also have "feelings," which can be assessed in other ways.

Some of these alterations and behavioral changes involve consciousness and association areas of the cerebral cortex.

With these aspects in mind, we can finally arrive at a definition of the limbic system as an interrelated group of cortical and subcortical structures that are involved in the regulation of the emotional state, with the accompanying behavioral, physiologic, and psychologic responses. The limbic system is connected with the rest of the brain. Unfortunately, the definition does not include one aspect of brain function that seems to have evolved in conjunction with the limbic system, *memory*.

Limbic functions can be summarized by the use of a rather simple mnemonic of five F's—feeding, fighting, fornicating, family, and forgetting. (In fact, remembering should be the fifth function but forgetting may be theoretically more correct as we shall see.)

In neuroanatomic terms, the limbic system now includes the following cortical and subcortical structures:

> *Cortical*—parts of the prefrontal and orbitofrontal cortex (the limbic forebrain), the cingulate gyrus, the parahippocampal gyrus, and some older cortical areas composing the hippocampal formation that are "buried" in the temporal lobe (in humans).

Subcortical—ventral portions of the striatum and pallidum, the basal forebrain, the amygdala, the septal region, parts of the thalamus, the hypothalamus, and portions of the midbrain (the limbic midbrain).

Included with these are the various tracts that interconnect the limbic structures. The olfactory system connects directly into the amygdala and certain limbic cortical areas.

Evolutionary Perspective

As in any field, many individuals have contributed to information and knowledge about the limbic system. In 1937, Dr. James Papez initiated the limbic era by proposing that a number of limbic structures in our brain formed the anatomic substratum for emotion. Three individuals extended our conceptual and factual understanding of the limbic system—Drs. Walle Nauta, Lennart Heimer, and Paul MacLean.

Dr. MacLean postulated that in fact three separable "brains" have evolved. The pre-mammalian (reptilian) brain has the capacity to look after the basic life functions and has organized ritualistic, stylized patterns of behavior. The forebrain structures, which relate to the external world (e.g., visual input), are adaptive, allowing for a modification of behavior, depending on the situation. MacLean suggested that the limbic system arises in early mammals to link these two brain functions; in some respects, the limbic system relates the reptilian brain, which monitors the internal milieu, with the newer forebrain areas (of mammals), which are responsible for analyzing the external environment.

It is thought that part of the function of the limbic system is to undo or unlock the fixed behavioral patterns of the old reptilian brain. To do this, one needs to "remember" what happened the last time when faced with a similar situation, hence the development of memory functions of the brain in association with the evolution of the limbic system. The availability of stored memories makes it possible for mammals to override or overrule the sterotypical behaviors of the reptile, allowing for more flexibility and adaptiveness when faced with a changing environment or altered circumstances. Therefore, we have listed the fifth F above as *forgetting* for the sake of the mnemonic, but this in fact has some theoretical basis.

It is also interesting to speculate that the development of the limbic system is closely associated with the development of self-awareness, or consciousness of the self.

FIGURE 70   # The Limbic Lobe

The cortical areas given the name *limbic* form a fringe (*limbus*) around the core structures of the diencephalon and midbrain. These cortical areas include the cingulate gyrus, the parahippocampal gyrus, and the cortical components found in the hippocampal formation.

The *cingulate gyrus* lies above the corpus callosum. MacLean's studies indicated that the development of this gyrus is correlated with the evolution of the mammalian species. He postulated that this gyrus is important for nursing and play behavior, characteristics associated in mammals with the rearing of young. It is this cluster of behavioral patterns that forms the basis for the fourth F in the list of functions of the limbic system, *family*.

If one follows the cingulate gyrus (and the corpus callosum) anteriorly (see Fig. 7), the cortical tissue bends around the rostrum of the callosum. Lying below this part of the corpus callosum are small cortical gyri that form part of the *septal region* (see Figs. 71 and 81). If one follows the cingulate gyrus posteriorly, the cortical tissue (via a narrow bridge) becomes continuous with the *parahippocampal gyrus*. This connection occurs via by a bundle of fibers in the white matter, known as the *cingulum bundle* (not shown), which connects the two areas reciprocally.

A number of cortical areas located in the most medial aspects of the temporal lobe, deep to the parahippocampal gyrus, form part of this "limbus"; these are collectively called the *hippocampal formation.* One of its major components, the *hippocampus proper,* is no longer found at the surface of the hemisphere, as would be expected for a cortical area. The explanation for this lies in the development of the region (discussed with Fig. 75). The other parts of the hippocampal formation are the *dentate gyrus,* part of which can be found at the surface, and the *subicular region,* a cortical region.

Some of these limbic cortical areas are structurally different than the typical six-layered neocortex that forms all the dorsolateral aspects of the hemispheres. The oldest cortical areas are found in the hippocampal formation—the hippocampus proper and the dentate cortex are three-layered cortical areas, and the subicular region has four or five layers (see Figs. 75 and 78). Not all parts of the cingulate gyrus are six-layered neocortex, though the parahippocampal gyrus is made up mostly of neocortical tissue (except most anteriorly).

Although the limbic lobe originally included only these cortical areas, other areas of the brain are now known to be involved in limbic functions, which has led to the use of the term *limbic system.* This includes large parts of the so-called prefrontal cortex, particularly cortical areas lying above the orbit, the *orbitofrontal cortex* (not labeled).

The *amygdala* (amygdaloid nucleus), as discussed earlier (see Fig. 12), is anatomically one of the basal ganglia. Functionally, and through its connections, it is part of the limbic system. Therefore, it is considered in this section of the *Atlas.* Other parts of the basal ganglia—namely, the ventral portions of the putamen and globus pallidus—may also have limbic functions (not shown on this diagram, see Figs. 82A and 82B).

Other subcortical areas now considered part of the limbic system are also shown in this diagram. These will be considered further in the next diagram, including some nuclei of the thalamus, parts of the hypothalamus (particularly the mammillary nuclei), and areas of the midbrain.

Of the many tracts of the limbic system, two major tracts have been included in this diagram—the fornix and the anterior commissure. The *fornix* is one of the more visible tracts and is often encountered during dissections of the brain (e.g., see Fig. 7). This fiber bundle connects the hippocampal formation with other subcortical areas. The *anterior commissure* is an older commissure than the corpus callosum and connects several structures of the limbic system on the two sides of the brain. These include the amygdala, the hippocampal formation, and parts of the parahippocampal gyrus. The anterior commissure will be seen on many of the limbic diagrams and is also a convenient reference point.

The details of the various limbic structures, the appropriate connections, and the functional aspects of these cortical and subcortical components of the limbic system are discussed with the appropriate diagrams.

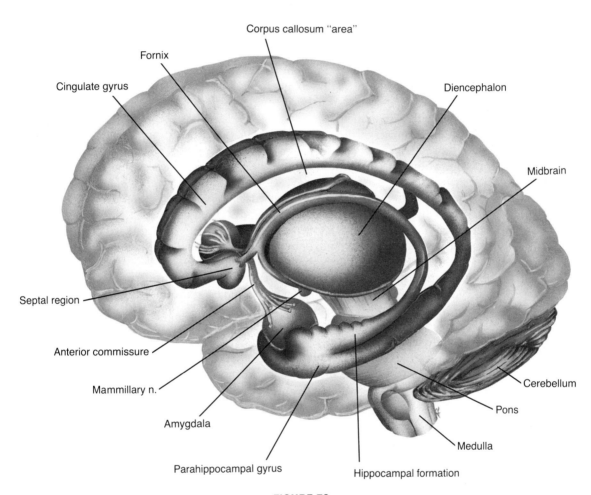

Corpus callosum "area"

Fornix

Cingulate gyrus

Diencephalon

Midbrain

Septal region

Anterior commissure

Mammillary n.

Amygdala

Cerebellum

Pons

Medulla

Parahippocampal gyrus

Hippocampal formation

FIGURE 70

179

FIGURE 71   # Diagram of the Limbic System

This is an overall diagram of both the cortical and subcortical components of the limbic system. Each of the structures, including the connections, is discussed in greater detail in subsequent illustrations. This diagram will be used as a "locator" map, where the parts of the limbic system being described are indicated appropriately (e.g., see Fig. 72). This locator diagram appears as an inset, while the major diagram presents the details of the structures being described.

The limbic system, as defined, consists of both cortical and subcortical structures. The cortical structures were reviewed in Figure 70 and are also represented in this diagram. They include the cingulate gyrus, the parahippocampal gyrus, and the older cortical areas of the hippocampal formation (the limbic lobe), as well as cortical areas of the frontal lobe.

The subcortical areas shown in this diagram include the amygdala, the septal region, some nuclei of the thalamus, the hypothalamus, and the limbic midbrain.

The *amygdala* is now considered a limbic structure. Again, parts of the ventral striatum and pallidum may have limbic functions.

The *septal region* includes two components—the cortical gyri below the rostrum of the corpus callosum and some nuclei deep to them. These nuclei are not located within the septum pellucidum in humans.

Two of the nuclei of the *thalamus,* the anterior group of nuclei and the dorsomedial nucleus (see Fig. 53), are part of the pathways of the limbic system, relaying information from subcortical nuclei to limbic parts of the cortex (the cingulate gyrus and areas of the prefrontal cortex).

The *hypothalamus* lies below and somewhat anterior to the thalamus. (The limits of the region are outlined in the inset diagram for Fig. 73.) Only a few of the nuclei are shown here, among them the prominent mammillary nucleus, which is visible on the inferior view of the brain (see Fig. 5). The connection of the hypothalamus to the pituitary gland is not shown.

The limbic system also includes parts of the *midbrain.* Some of the descending limbic pathways terminate in this region, and it is important to consider the role of this area in limbic functions. Both the septal region on one side and the midbrain on the other are not really far from the hypothalamus.

The *olfactory system* is described with the limbic system, since many of its connections are directly with limbic areas. Years ago, it was commonplace to think of various limbic structures as part of the "smell brain," the *rhinencephalon.* We now know that this is to a large part incorrect and that the limbic system has many other functional capabilities.

Not represented in this diagram is the region known as the *basal forebrain area.* This is a subcortical region, which is composed of a group of structures located beside the hypothalamus and below the anterior commissure (see Figs. 82A and 82B). This somewhat obscure region has connections with limbic areas, particularly prefrontal cortex, and may play a major role in human emotionality.

The various pathways shown are discussed at the appropriate time with the relevant structures.

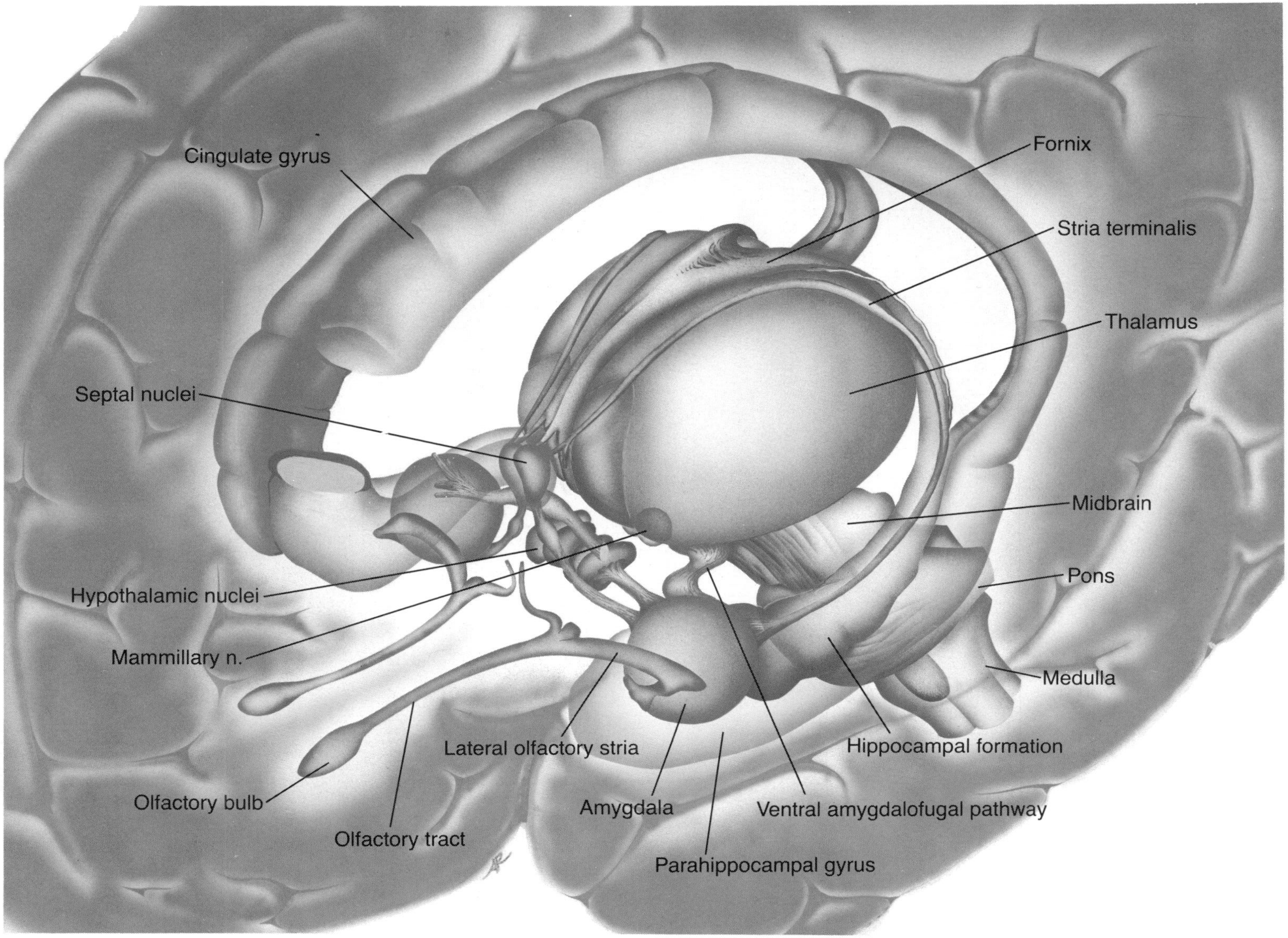

Fornix

Stria terminalis

Thalamus

Midbrain

Pons

Medulla

Hippocampal formation

Ventral amygdalofugal pathway

Parahippocampal gyrus

Amygdala

Lateral olfactory stria

Olfactory tract

Olfactory bulb

Mammillary n.

Hypothalamic nuclei

Septal nuclei

Cingulate gyrus

FIGURE 71

181

FIGURE 72 **Amygdala**

LIMBIC DIAGRAM (INSET)

The amygdala is a subcortical nuclear structure located in the temporal lobe in humans. As a subcortical nucleus of the forebrain, it belongs by definition with the basal ganglia but, because of its connections, is usually described with the limbic system. The amygdala is located between the temporal pole and the "end" of the inferior horn of the lateral ventricle (in the temporal lobe; see Figs. 13 and 76). Its mass is responsible for the elevation known as the *uncus,* which is seen on the inferior aspect of the brain (see Figs. 4 and 5). Two fiber tracts are shown connecting the amygdala to other limbic structures—a dorsal one (the stria terminalis) and a ventral one (the ventral amygdalofugal pathway, consisting of two parts).

CONNECTIONS AND FUNCTIONS

One of the major differences between the amygdala and the other parts of the basal ganglia is that the amygdala is not a homogeneous nuclear structure but is composed of different component parts. (These are not usually studied in an introductory course.)

The amygdala receives a variety of inputs from other parts of the brain, including the adjacent parahippocampal gyrus (not illustrated). It receives olfactory input directly (via the lateral olfactory stria; see Fig. 81), and indirectly from the cortex of the uncal region (as shown on the left side of the diagram).

The amygdaloid nuclei are connected to the hypothalamus, thalamus (mainly the dorsomedial nucleus; see Fig. 80), and the septal region. These connections, which are reciprocal, travel through two routes (seen also in the inset):

> *Dorsal route:* Known as the *stria terminalis,* this pathway follows the ventricular curve and is found on the upper aspect of the thalamus (see Figs. 74 and 76). (The stria terminalis lies adjacent to the body of the caudate nucleus in this location.)
> *Ventral route:* Known as the ventral pathway or *ventral amygdalofugal pathway,* this route, which goes through the basal forebrain region (see Fig. 82A), connects to the hypothalamus (as shown) and to the thalamus (the fibers are shown en route).

Further possible connections of the amygdala with other limbic structures can occur via the hypothalamus (discussed with that structure; see Fig. 73), the septal region (see Fig. 74), or the dorsomedial nucleus of the thalamus (see Fig. 80). The anterior commissure conveys connections between the nuclei of the two sides. The amygdala also has connections with autonomic-related nuclei in the midbrain (the limbic midbrain), and possibly also in the medulla. These influences may be direct or indirect (as shown).

Functionally, stimulation of the amygdaloid nucleus produces a variety of vegetative responses, including licking and chewing movements. In animal experimentation, stimulation of the amygdala produces a "rage" response, whereas removal of the amygdala (bilaterally) results in docility. Bilateral removal of the anterior parts of the temporal lobe (including the amygdala) in monkeys produces a number of effects collectively called the *Klüver-Bucy syndrome.* The monkeys became tamer after surgery, put everything into their mouths, and displayed inappropriate sexual behavior.

In rather unusual circumstances, bilateral destruction of the amygdala is recommended in humans for individuals (particularly those in institutions) whose violent behavior cannot be controlled by other means. This type of treatment is called *psychosurgery.*

The amygdala has a low threshold for electrical discharges, which may make it prone to be the focus for the development of seizures. These may be accompanied by the vegetative responses mentioned previously. An experimental model of epilepsy, called *kindling,* may be triggered in the amygdala because of its low electrical threshold. The amygdala also contains a high amount of enkephalins.

The role of the amygdala in the formation of memory is not clear. Bilateral removal of the anterior portions of the temporal lobe in humans, for the treatment of severe cases of epilepsy, results in a memory disorder, which is described with the hippocampal formation (see Figs. 75 and 77). It is possible that the role of the amygdala in the formation of memories is mediated either through the connections of this nuclear complex with the hippocampal formation, or with the dorsomedial nucleus of the thalamus, or both.

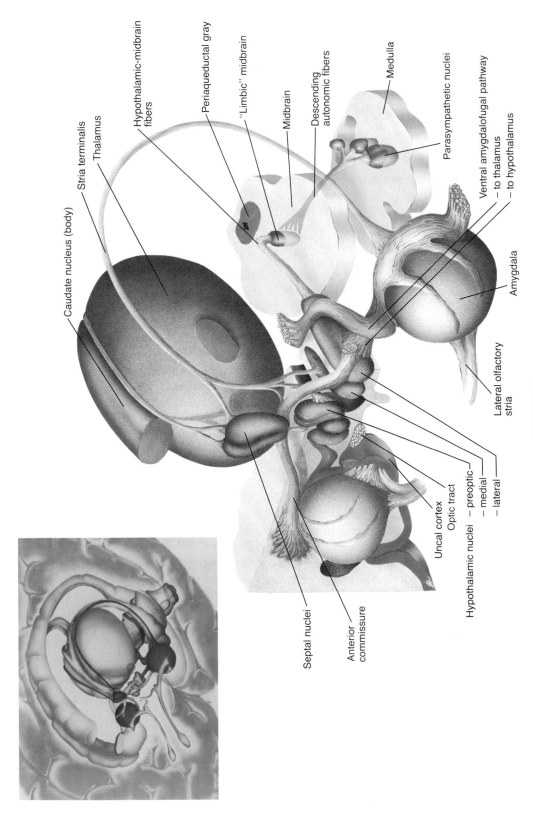

Caudate nucleus (body)

Stria terminalis

Thalamus

Hypothalamic-midbrain fibers

Periaqueductal gray

"Limbic" midbrain

Midbrain

Descending autonomic fibers

Medulla

Parasympathetic nuclei

Ventral amygdalofugal pathway
– to thalamus
– to hypothalamus

Amygdala

Lateral olfactory stria

Uncal cortex
Optic tract
Hypothalamic nuclei – preoptic
– medial
– lateral

Anterior commissure

Septal nuclei

FIGURE 72

183

FIGURE 73

Hypothalamus, Septal Region, and Limbic Midbrain

LIMBIC DIAGRAM (INSET)

This diagram of the limbic system focuses on the hypothalamic region (see Fig. 7). The hypothalamic area is outlined, and some of its nuclear parts are shown (on each side)—a lateral and a medial group of nuclei and the mammillary nuclei. The hypothalamus is closely connected to the septal region (not marked; to be discussed in the next diagram). It is also connected directly with areas of the midbrain, which are collectively called the *limbic midbrain*. There are also some indirect connections to nuclei of the medulla via descending autonomic fibers. Both parts of the brain stem are therefore included in this illustration.

Hypothalamus

The hypothalamus is primarily responsible for the control of homeostatic mechanisms, including water balance, temperature regulation, and food intake. It accomplishes these tasks in two ways—as a neural structure linked into the limbic system and as a neuroendocrine structure controlling the activities of the pituitary gland. In its neural role, it acts as the "head ganglion" of the autonomic nervous system, influencing both sympathetic and parasympathetic activities.

Some of the major inputs to the hypothalamus come from limbic structures, including the amygdala (via the stria terminalis and the ventral pathway; see Fig. 72) and the hippocampal formation (via the fornix; see Fig. 75). Stimulation of particular small areas of the hypothalamus can lead to a variety of behaviors (e.g., sham rage), similar to that which occurs following stimulation of other parts of the limbic system (e.g., the amygdala).

The diagram divides the hypothalamic nuclei into a medial and a lateral group, with the third ventricle between the two sides. A number of nuclei that control the anterior pituitary gland are located in the medial group and also in the preoptic nuclei (shown in the previous diagram). This control system occurs via the median eminence (see Fig. 5) and the portal system of veins along the pituitary stalk. Other nuclei in the supraoptic region connect directly (via axons) with the posterior pituitary. The hypothalamus is also connected with the midbrain by means of a fiber bundle (labeled in the previous diagram—the hypothalamic–midbrain fibers).

The mammillary nuclei are of special importance as part of the limbic system. They receive a direct input from the hippocampal formation (via the fornix) and give rise to fibers that connect directly to the limbic midbrain, the *mammillotegmental tract*. In addition, a major fiber tract, the *mammillothalamic tract*, connects the mammillary nuclei with the thalamic anterior group of nuclei (see Fig. 53), part of the limbic diencephalon.

Running through the lateral mass of the hypothalamus is a prominent fiber tract, the *medial forebrain bundle*. This interconnects the hypothalamus reciprocally with two areas—the septal region of the forebrain and the limbic midbrain.

Septal Region

This region includes the cortical areas under the rostrum of the corpus callosum (subcallosal gyrus) and nuclei deep to this area. (The septal region is discussed with the next diagram.) The medial forebrain bundle connects the septal region with the hypothalamus and the limbic midbrain, reciprocally. The septal region also has another connecting pathway with the midbrain, which is shown in the next diagram.

Limbic Midbrain

A number of limbic pathways terminate within the reticular formation of the midbrain (see Fig. 49, including the periaqueductal gray), leading to the inclusion of this area in discussion of the structures that make up the limbic system and to the use of the term *limbic midbrain*. Five pathways terminate within the limbic midbrain, three of which are shown in this diagram (the medial forebrain bundle, the mammillotegmental tract, and the dorsal longitudinal bundle; (not labeled) the hypothalamic-midbrain fibers were shown in Fig. 72, and the habenulointerpeduncular tract is described in Fig. 74.

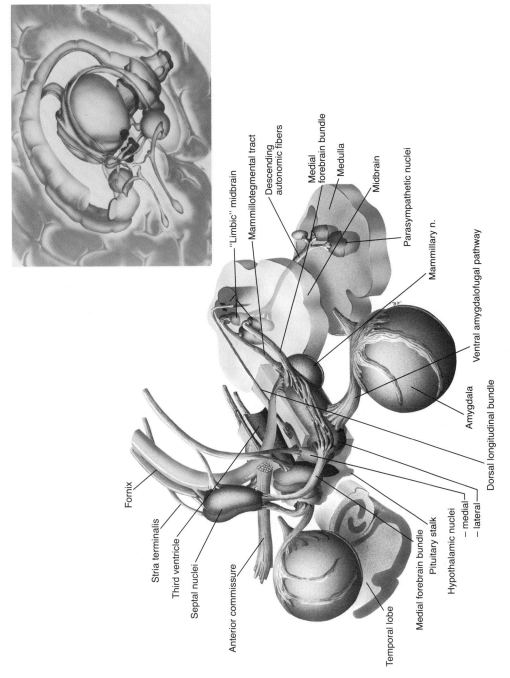

Fornix

Stria terminalis

Third ventricle

Septal nuclei

Anterior commissure

Temporal lobe

Medial forebrain bundle

Pituitary stalk

Hypothalamic nuclei
– medial
– lateral

Dorsal longitudinal bundle

Amygdala

Ventral amygdalofugal pathway

Mammillary n.

Parasympathetic nuclei

Midbrain

Medulla

Medial forebrain bundle

Descending autonomic fibers

Mammillotegmental tract

"Limbic" midbrain

FIGURE 73

185

FIGURE 74   # Septal Region, Habenula, and Limbic Midbrain

LIMBIC DIAGRAM (INSET)

The limbic structures being considered in this diagram are the septal region, both cortical and nuclear parts, and a region at the posterior end of the diencephalon, the habenula. From here, fibers are sent to the midbrain region, the limbic midbrain. Two tracts are associated with this pathway—the stria medullaris from septal region to habenula, and the habenulointerpeduncular tract to the midbrain (seen in the main diagram). The pineal gland is seen attached at the posterior margin of the diencephalon, just behind the habenular nuclei.

Septal Region

The septal region includes both cortical and subcortical areas that belong to the forebrain. The cortical areas are found under the rostrum of the corpus callosum and include the *subcallosal gyrus* (see Figs. 7, 70, and 81). Nuclei lying deep in this region are called the *septal nuclei* and in some species (not humans) are in fact located within the septum pellucidum (the septum that separates the bodies of the lateral ventricles).

Rats with small electrodes implanted in their septal regions quickly learn to press a bar that completes an electrical circuit and sends a tiny (harmless) electric current through the brain tissue. In fact, they press the bar virtually nonstop! From this, it was inferred that the animals derive some type of pleasant "sensation" from stimulation of this region—hence its nickname, the "pleasure center." Similar behavior can be produced using other areas, but this type of positive effect is not seen in all parts of the brain, and an opposite (negative) reaction is seen in some areas.

The septal region receives input from the amygdala (via the stria terminalis; see Fig. 72) and the hippocampal formation (via the fornix; see Fig. 75). The stria terminalis, which lies on the dorsal aspect of the thalamus, is also shown in this diagram. It is located beside the body of the caudate nucleus, situated above the diencephalon (see Figs. 53 and 76). The medial forebrain bundle, shown in the previous diagram, connects the septal region with the hypothalamus and the limbic midbrain. All these connections are reciprocal.

Habenula

The habenular nuclei are a group of small nuclei that are part of the diencephalon. They are situated at the posterior end of the thalamus, on its upper surface.

There is another circuit whereby septal influences are conveyed to the midbrain. The first part of the pathway is the *stria medullaris,* which connects the septal nuclei (region) with the habenular nuclei. The stria medullaris is found on the medial surface of the thalamus. (The tract is seen in Fig. 7, a view of the medial aspect of the brain. It is not labeled but can be located above the letter T on the diagram.) The diagram shows one diencephalon (mainly the thalamus), with the stria medullaris on its medial aspect. Some fibers of the stria come from nuclei of the hypothalamus known as the preoptic region.

From the habenular nuclei, a tract descends to the midbrain reticular formation, mainly to a nucleus located between the cerebral peduncles, the *interpeduncular nucleus* (see cross section B2 in Fig. 29). This tract is best called the *habenulointerpeduncular tract.* (In some texts, it is labeled the fasciculus retroflexus.) The further connections of the interpeduncular nucleus are unclear but are thought to be similar to those of other midbrain reticular formation nuclei that have a limbic function.

Limbic Midbrain

From the limbic midbrain, descending autonomic pathways (see Fig. 73) apparently convey the information to the parasympathetic and other nuclei of the pons and medulla (e.g., the dorsal motor nucleus of the vagus, the facial nucleus for emotional facial responses), as well as to areas of the reticular formation of the medulla concerned with cardiovascular and respiratory control mechanisms (discussed with Fig. 25). Other connections are apparently made with autonomic neurons in the spinal cord (e.g., for sympathetic-type responses).

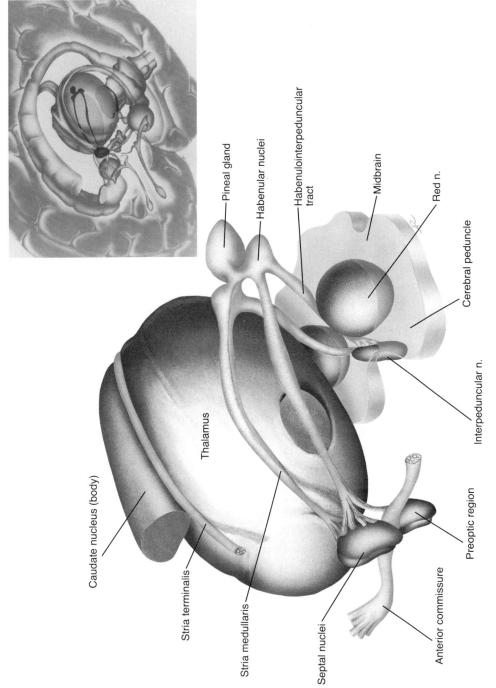

Caudate nucleus (body)

Thalamus

Stria terminalis

Pineal gland

Habenular nuclei

Habenulointerpeduncular tract

Midbrain

Red n.

Cerebral peduncle

Interpeduncular n.

Stria medullaris

Septal nuclei

Preoptic region

Anterior commissure

FIGURE 74

FIGURE 75   # Hippocampal Formation

LIMBIC DIAGRAM (INSET)

Much of the difficulty of understanding the structures of the hippocampal formation in humans is their anatomic location deep within the medial portions of the temporal lobe. In the rat, the hippocampal formation is located dorsally, above the thalamus. During the evolution of the temporal lobe, these structures were pulled into the temporal lobe, leaving behind a fiber pathway, the *fornix,* which is located above the thalamus. (In fact, a vestigial part of the hippocampal formation is still located above the corpus callosum, as shown in this illustration.) The fornix connects with the septal region and mammillary nuclei. In the temporal lobe, the hippocampal formation is adjacent to the six-layered parahippocampal gyrus, with which it has extensive connections.

Hippocampus Proper, Dentate Gyrus, and Subiculum

One expects a cortical area to be found at the surface of the brain (even if this surface is located deep within a fissure). The hippocampal formation includes three cortical areas—the hippocampus proper, the dentate gyrus, and the subicular region. These structures are included in the description of the limbic "lobe" (see Fig. 70). During the evolution and development of the hippocampal formation, these areas become rolled up inside the brain. (The student should consult Williams and Warwick, one of the reference books listed in the Annotated Bibliography, for a detailed understanding of this phenomenon.) Of the three, the hippocampus proper is found completely within the brain. All of these areas are older-type cortices consisting of fewer than six layers.

The hippocampal formation is probably the most important part of the limbic system and certainly the most complex. This structure probably has the critical function in the formation of new memories.

HIPPOCAMPUS PROPER

The hippocampus proper consists of a three-layered cortical area. This forms a large mass, which actually intrudes into the ventricular space of the inferior horn of the lateral ventricle (see Figs. 77 and 78). The cortical region has been divided into a number of subportions (usually studied in more advanced courses). In a microscopic section cut in the transverse plane through this region, the hippocampus proper takes the shape of a seahorse. It is from this shape that the name *hippocampus* is derived, from the French word for seahorse. The other name for this area is *Ammon's horn.*

DENTATE GYRUS

The dentate gyrus is also a phylogenetically older cortical area consisting of only three layers. During the formation discussed above, the leading edge of the cortex detaches itself and becomes the dentate gyrus. Parts of it remain visible at the surface of the brain. Since this small surface is buried on the most medial aspect of the temporal lobe and is located deep within a fissure, it is rarely found in studies of the gross brain. Once visualized, it is seen to have ridges or a serrated surface, which seemed to suggest tooth marks, giving it the name *dentate* (referring to teeth).

The dentate gyrus is shown on the view of the medial aspect of the temporal lobe (on the far side of the illustration). A section through the temporal lobe (as seen in the lower part of the diagram) indicates that the dentate gyrus is more extensive than its visible medial portion.

SUBICULAR REGION

The next part of the cortically rolled-in structures that make up the hippocampal formation is the subicular region (see also Fig. 78). The cortical thickness is transitional, starting from the three-layered hippocampal formation and increasing to the six-layered parahippocampal gyrus. (Again, there are a number of subparts of this area that are rarely studied in an introductory course.)

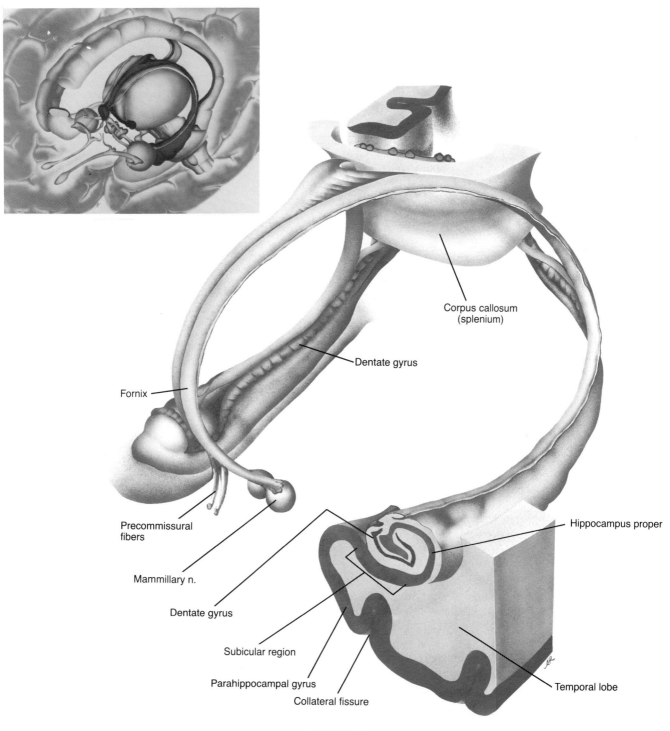

Corpus callosum
(splenium)

Dentate gyrus

Fornix

Precommissural
fibers

Mammillary n.

Dentate gyrus

Subicular region

Parahippocampal gyrus

Collateral fissure

Hippocampus proper

Temporal lobe

FIGURE 75

FIGURE 76 # Limbic Structures and the Lateral Ventricle

During the development of the temporal lobe, a number of structures are pulled into it—the lateral ventricle, the hippocampal formation, and the caudate nucleus, as well as various tracts, the fornix, and stria terminalis. Many of the structures follow the inner curvature of the ventricle, which means that they are situated in the lower aspect of the ventricle above the thalamus, and on the upper aspect of the ventricle in the temporal lobe.

This view of the relationship of these various structures is augmented by a number of sections at various points:

1   The first section is through the anterior horn of the ventricle, in front of the interventricular foramen (foramen of Monro).
2   The following section is over the dorsal aspect of the thalamus and above the third ventricle.
3   The third section shows the ventricle at its curvature, into the temporal lobe.
4   The last section is through the temporal lobe, including the hippocampal formation.

FORNIX

The fornix is easily found in studies of the gross brain (e.g., Fig. 7). Its fibers, which course on the inner aspect of the ventricle as they sweep forward above the thalamus, can be seen as a continuation of the hippocampal formation (see Figs. 75 and 77). In the area above the thalamus and below the corpus callosum (see Fig. 78), the fornix is found at the lower edge of the septum pellucidum. Here, the fornix of one side is in fact adjacent to that of the other side (see also Fig. 71). There may be interconnections between the two sides in this area.

The fibers of the fornix pass in front of the interventricular formen (see medial view of brain in Fig. 7). At this point, some of the fibers are given off to the septal region and pass in front of the anterior commissure; these are the *precommissural fibers* (see Fig. 75). Others continue (behind the anterior commissure) through the hypothalamus and terminate in the mammillary nucleus (which is not portrayed in this diagram; see Fig. 55).

STRIA TERMINALIS

The stria terminalis (connecting the amygdala with the septal region and hypothalamus) follows essentially the same course as the fornix. Its fibers lie slightly more medially and are found on the dorsal aspect of the thalamus, in the floor of the body of the lateral ventricle. In the temporal lobe, the stria is found in the roof of the inferior horn of the lateral ventricle (see Fig. 55).

CAUDATE NUCLEUS

The various parts of the caudate nucleus are shown in this diagram (see Fig. 13). The large head is found in relation to the anterior horn of the lateral ventricle, into which it bulges. This is also seen in a horizontal section through the brain (see Fig. 18). The body of the caudate nucleus is coincident with the body of the lateral ventricle, being found on its lateral aspect (see Figs. 13 and 55). In this location, it is situated above the thalamus (see Figs. 72 and 74).

As the caudate nucleus curves into the temporal lobe, it becomes the tail of the caudate nucleus. In the temporal lobe, it is found on the upper aspect of the inferior horn of the ventricle, its roof (see Figs. 13 and 55).

The amygdala is clearly seen to be situated anterior to the temporal horn of the lateral ventricle and in front of the hippocampal formation (see Fig. 70).

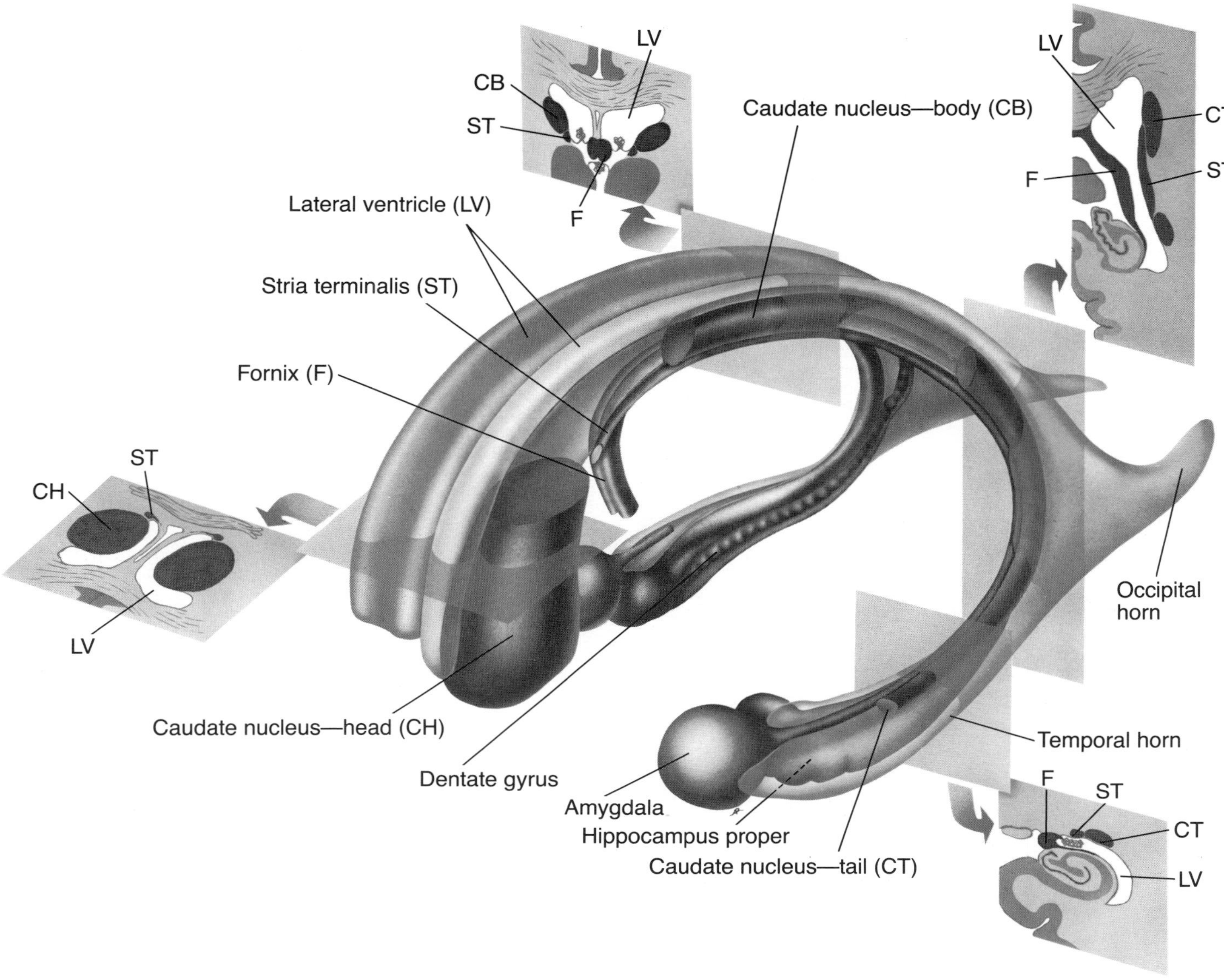

CT
ST
LV
F

Caudate nucleus—body (CB)

LV
CB
ST
F

Caudate nucleus

Lateral ventricle (LV)

Stria terminalis (ST)

Fornix (F)

ST
CH
LV

Caudate nucleus—head (CH)

Dentate gyrus

Amygdala
Hippocampus proper
Caudate nucleus—tail (CT)

Temporal horn

Occipital
horn

ST
CT
F
LV

FIGURE 76

191

FIGURE 77   # Hippocampus (Photographic View)

The brain is shown from the dorsolateral aspect. The left hemisphere is partially obscured by the gloved hand holding the structures.

The right hemisphere has been dissected by removing some cortical tissue of the temporal lobe and exposing the inferior horn of the lateral ventricle (see Fig. 10A). This dissection exposes a large mass of tissue (see Figs. 70, 71, and 75) which is in fact protruding into this part of the ventricle, the "hippocampus." The protrusion of the hippocampus into the inferior horn of the lateral ventricle can be seen in coronal sections through this region (see Figs. 19, 76, and 78). The choroid plexus tissue has been removed from this part of the ventricle to improve visualization of the structures.

In a gross brain dissection, it is not possible to refer precisely to the portions of the hippocampal formation. Having reviewed the hippocampal formation in previous diagrams, it is mainly the hippocampus proper, with the dentate gyrus, that forms this large mass of tissue.

The fornix, the fiber bundle that arises from the visible "hippocampus," can be identified on its uppermost aspect. The fornix receives fibers from the hippocampus proper and the subicular region. This fiber bundle continues from the hippocampal formation and sweeps over the top of the thalamus (see Figs. 70 and 71). As seen on coronal sections, the fornix is "attached" to the undersurface of the corpus callosum (see Figs. 19 and 78).

CONNECTIONS AND FUNCTION

The hippocampal formation receives its major input from the adjacent parahippocampal gyrus as well as the amygdala. There are extensive interconnections within the component parts of the hippocampal formation itself.

Part of the output of this cortical region is directed back toward the parahippocampal gyrus, which itself has extensive connections with other cortical areas of the brain, particularly sensory areas. This is analogous to the cortical association pathways described earlier. The other major output of the hippocampal formation is through the fornix. Only the hippocampus proper and the subicular region project fibers into the fornix. This can be regarded as a subcortical pathway that terminates in the septal region (see Figs. 73 and 75; via the precommissural fibers) and in the mammillary nucleus of the hypothalamus (see Figs. 70 and 75). Undoubtedly, there are also reciprocal connections in the fornix. The dentate gyrus only connects with other parts of the hippocampal formation and does not project beyond.

Recent studies in humans indicate that one portion of the hippocampal formation is the critical structure for the formation of new memories. This means that for the brain to "remember" something, new information must be registered within the hippocampal formation, possibly involving the parahippocampal gyrus. This information is "processed" by these structures, which retain it for a brief time. For it to be remembered for longer periods, something occurs so that the transient memory trace is transferred to other parts of the brain and stored as a long-term memory trace. (An analogy to computers may be useful here.)

Bilateral damage or removal of the anterior temporal lobe structures, including the amygdala and the hippocampal formation, leads to a unique condition in which the person can no longer form new memories, although old memories are intact. The individual cannot remember what occurred moments after the event. Therefore, he or she is not able to learn—that is, to acquire new information—and is unable to function independently. The literature reports on a patient known as H.M. who was reduced to such a state when surgeons inadvertently removed the medial temporal structures (for intractable epilepsy), without knowing that the contralateral structures were damaged. He has been extensively studied by neuropsychologists. Now that it is known what may occur with surgery in this region, special testing is done to ascertain that the side contralateral to the surgery is intact and functioning. Damage to this area, termed *medial temporal sclerosis,* occurs as the result of a variety of conditions.

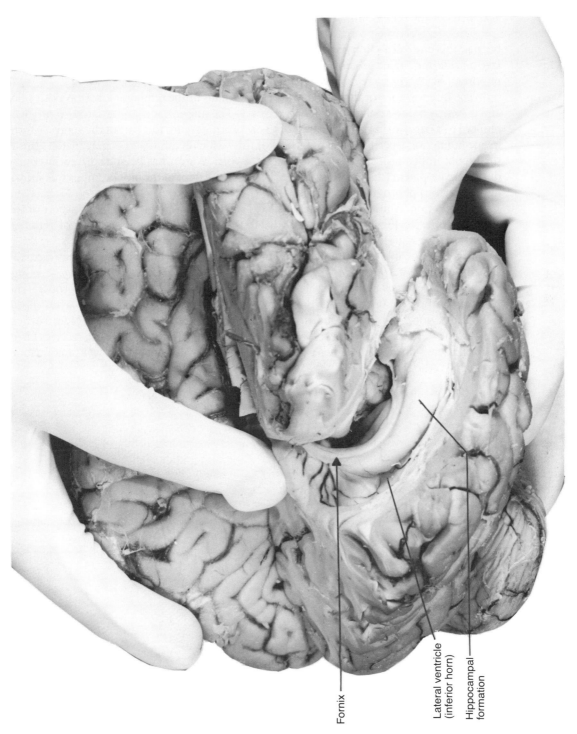

Fornix

Lateral ventricle
(inferior horn)

Hippocampal
formation

FIGURE 77

193

FIGURE 78

Coronal Brain Section (Photographic View)

This section is taken posterior to the one shown in Figure 19. The basal ganglia are no longer present. The most posterior portions of the thalamus, the *pulvinar*, are seen, inferior to the lateral ventricles. Between the thalamus and the corpus callosum is the fornix. The section also includes the brain stem.

The space between the thalamic areas shown (the pulvinar) is not the third ventricle because this coronal section has been taken so posteriorly (see Fig. 53). The large space is in fact outside the brain, posterior to the diencephalic region (see Fig. 7). It contains some important veins that were removed from this specimen.

The inferior horn of the lateral ventricles is found in the temporal lobes on both sides and is seen as only a small crescent-shaped cavity. The inferior horn of the lateral ventricle is reduced to a narrow slit because a mass of tissue protrudes into this part of the ventricle from its medioinferior aspect. Closer inspection of this tissue reveals that it is gray matter; this is the hippocampus proper. The hippocampus, a cortical area, has been displaced internally during development (discussed with Fig. 75). The full extent of the hippocampus was shown in the previous photograph.

This section includes the collateral sulcus, seen previously on the inferior aspect of the temporal lobe (see Fig. 4). The gyrus medial to this sulcus is the parahippocampal gyrus, so named because it lies beside the "hippocampus" (see Figs. 70 and 71).

It is also possible to follow the gray matter from the parahippocampal gyrus medially and through an intermediate zone, known as the *subiculum* or the *subicular region* (see Fig. 75), until it becomes continuous with the gray matter of the hippocampus proper. The parahippocampal gyrus is a six-layered cortex. This is reduced to four or five layers in the subicular region. The hippocampus proper has only three layers and is an older cortical region. The subicular region forms part of the hippocampal formation; it both receives fibers from and sends fibers to the other parts of the hippocampal formation, as well as contributing fibers to the fornix.

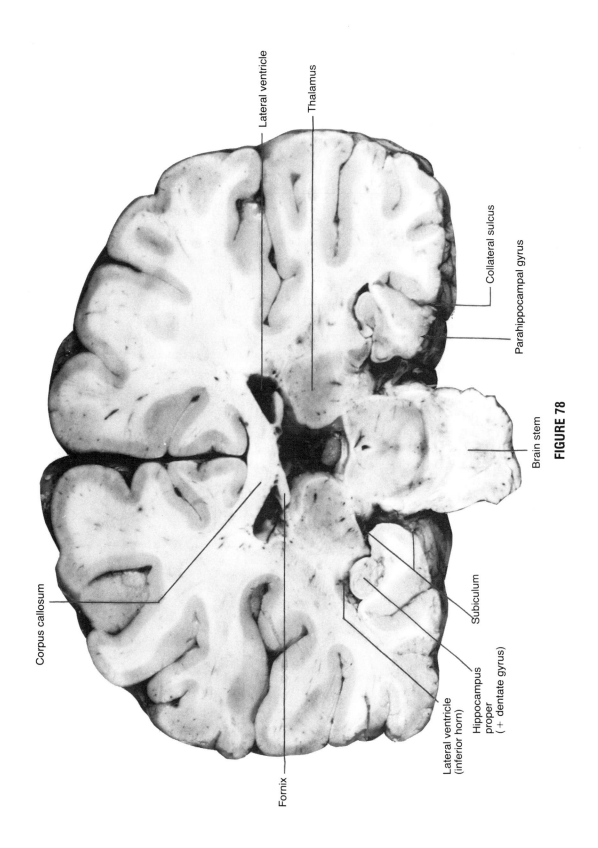

Lateral ventricle

Thalamus

Collateral sulcus

Parahippocampal gyrus

Corpus callosum

Brain stem

Subiculum

Fornix

Lateral ventricle
(inferior horn)

Hippocampus
proper
(+ dentate gyrus)

FIGURE 78

195

FIGURE 79   # Limbic Diencephalon: Anterior Nucleus

LIMBIC DIAGRAM (INSET)

This diagram of the structures of the limbic system has certain parts accentuated, since these are the areas shown in the detailed diagram. The thalamus on the far side is the one seen in the detailed diagram, as are the two mammillary nuclei and a small piece of the cingulate gyrus.

ANTERIOR THALAMIC NUCLEUS—CINGULATE GYRUS

The projection from the hippocampal formation courses in the fornix and terminates in part in the mammillary nuclei. From here, the *mammillothalamic tract* (see Fig. 53) ascends to the anterior group of thalamic nuclei (see Fig. 80, not labeled).

Axons leave the anterior nuclei of the thalamus and course through the anterior limb of the internal capsule. These fibers course between the caudate nucleus (head and body) and the lentiform nucleus (which is just visible in the backgroun). The axons terminate in the cortex of the *cingulate gyrus* after passing through the corpus callosum.

This pathway is part of a circuit described by J. Papez about 50 years ago. He proposed that this set of structures was responsible for the subjective emotional experience. As originally proposed, the hippocampus transmitted its information to the *mammillary nuclei* of the hypothalamus by means of the fornix; the information was then relayed to the *anterior nuclei* of the thalamus, and then to the *cingulate gyrus*. This gyrus is known to be reciprocally connected to the parahippocampal gyrus (by an association bundle called the *cingulum*). The precise functional significance of this circuit, known as the *Papez circuit,* has not yet been clearly elucidated. It is now known that the parahippocampal gyrus and the hippocampal formation have extensive interconnections.

In the days of psychosurgery, bilateral removal of the cingulate gyrus was performed for certain psychiatric disorders, including extreme obsessive-compulsive behavior. This type of surgery is rarely performed now because new and powerful drugs have been found to help treat these disorders of humankind.

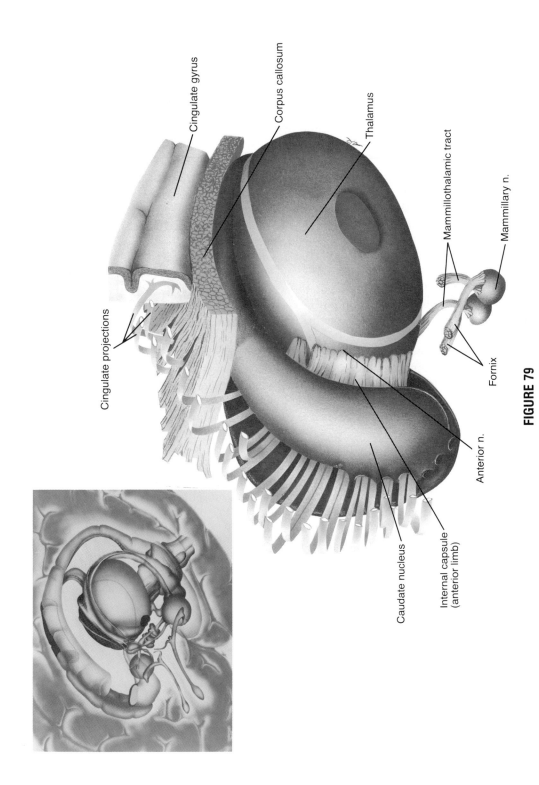

Cingulate gyrus

Corpus callosum

Thalamus

Mammillothalamic tract

Mammillary n.

Cingulate projections

Fornix

Anterior n.

Caudate nucleus

Internal capsule
(anterior limb)

FIGURE 79

FIGURE 80

Limbic Diencephalon: Dorsomedial Nucleus

LIMBIC DIAGRAM (INSET)

As in Figure 79, the areas indicated are those that are shown in the more detailed diagram. These areas include the thalamus on the distal side, as well as the thalamus situated nearer the viewer. The nearer thalamus is represented differently since it is sectioned in the detailed drawing. Also represented is the cortex of the frontal lobe (prefrontal cortex).

DORSOMEDIAL NUCLEUS—PREFRONTAL CORTEX

The dorsomedial nucleus of the thalamus, an association nucleus (see Fig. 53), collects information from a variety of sources. Some comes from the amygdala via the ventral pathway (see Fig. 72), and other information comes from other thalamic nuclei. It also collects information from various hypothalamic nuclei, as well as the ventral parts of the basal ganglia that are connected with the limbic system (see Fig. 82A).

The dorsomedial nucleus projects heavily to the prefrontal cortex, the cortex of the frontal lobe that lies in front of the various motor areas and that also extends onto the medial and inferior surfaces of the brain (see Figs. 2, 4, and 7). This is a reciprocal connection. The course of the fibers through the anterior limb of the internal capsule (between the head of the caudate nucleus and the lentiform nucleus) is seen on the left side of the diagram.

The functional aspect of this connection has been extensively studied in humans, because surgical interruption of these fibers (bilaterally) used to be done frequently as psychosurgery for some psychiatric disorders, including schizophrenia. The operation is called a *frontal lobotomy*. Bilateral sectioning of this frontal projection pathway results in profound personality changes. The person becomes emotionally "flat" and loses some hard-to-define human quality in his or her interpersonal interactions. In addition, a lobotomized individual may perform socially inappropriate acts that are not in keeping with his or her personality before the surgery. "Intelligence" does not seem to be affected. Today, other forms of treatment are available, particularly medications, and the surgery is rarely performed.

Frontal lobotomy may, however, still be recommended for the treatment of pain in terminally ill cancer patients. After the surgery, the individual still has the pain but no longer "suffers" from it; that is, the psychic aspect of the pain has been removed. There may even be a reduced demand for pain medication such as morphine. Thus, lobotomy can be seen as a part of the palliative care of an individual.

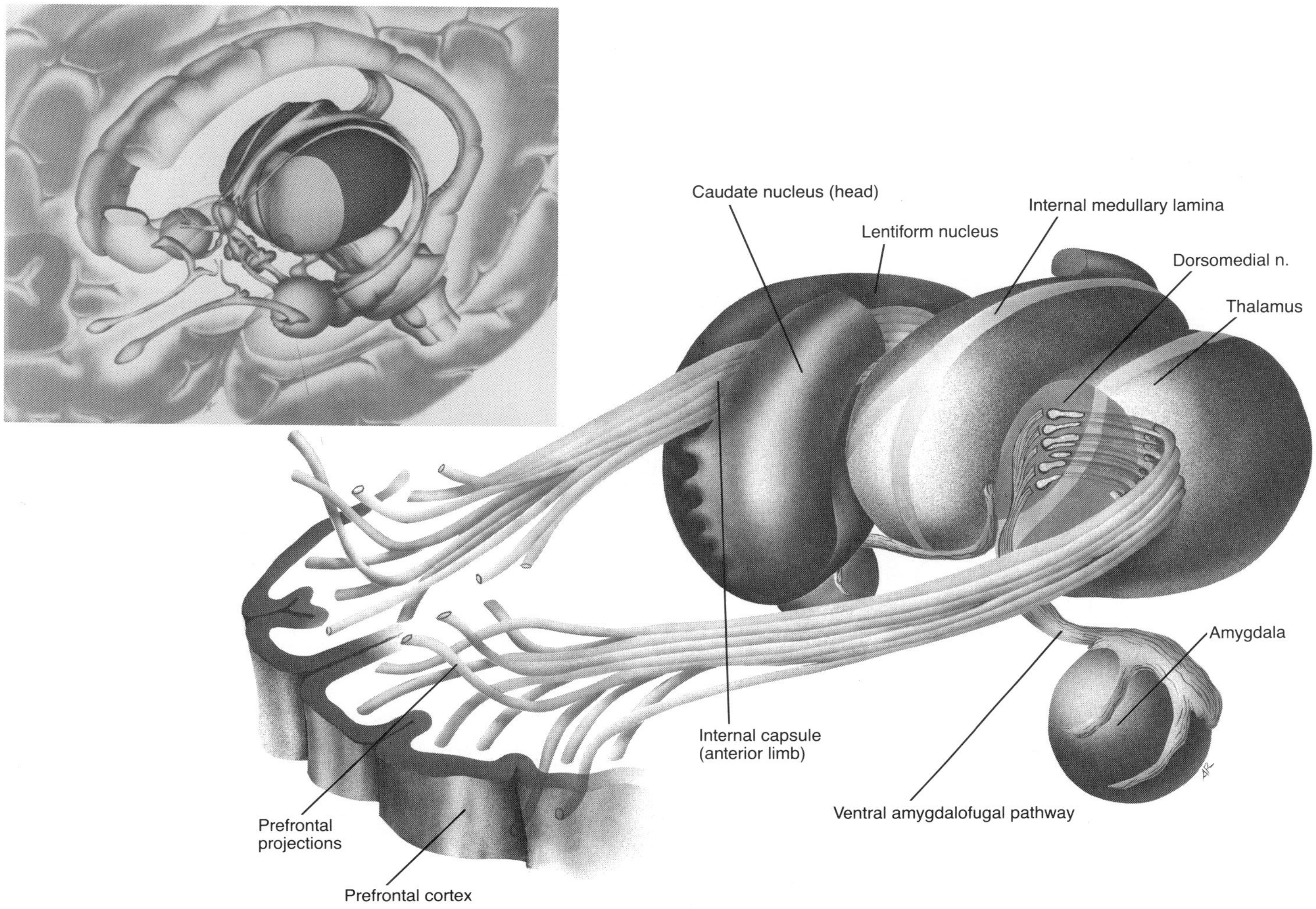

Internal medullary lamina

Dorsomedial n.

Thalamus

Amygdala

Lentiform nucleus

Caudate nucleus (head)

Ventral amygdalofugal pathway

Internal capsule (anterior limb)

Prefrontal cortex

Prefrontal projections

FIGURE 80

199

FIGURE 81   # Olfactory System

OLFACTORY STRUCTURES (INSET)

The olfactory system, which governs the sense of smell, is a phylogenetically older sensory system. This sensory system sends information directly into the limbic system, without a relay nucleus in the thalamus. Its size depends somewhat on the species, being larger in animals with more highly developed senses of smell. In humans, the olfactory system is small. Its component parts are the olfactory bulb and tract, which are located on the inferior surface of the frontal lobes, and various areas where the primary olfactory fibers terminate, including the amygdala and the cortex over the uncal region.

OLFACTORY BULB AND TRACT

The sensory cells in the nasal mucosa project their axons into the olfactory bulb. These tiny fibers, which constitute the actual peripheral *olfactory nerve* (CN I), pierce the cribriform plate in the roof of the nose. There is a complex series of interactions in the *olfactory bulb,* and one of the cells then projects its axon into the *olfactory tract.* The olfactory bulb and tract are therefore part of the CNS.

The olfactory tract runs posteriorly along the inferior surface of the frontal lobe (see Figs. 4 and 5) and terminates, apparently, by dividing into *lateral and medial tracts,* called *stria.* At this dividing point, there are a number of small holes for the entry of several blood vessels to the interior of the brain, the striate arteries (see Figs. 82A and 82B); this triangular area is known as the *anterior perforated space.*

Associated with the olfactory tract is another nucleus, the *anterior olfactory nucleus* (not shown), which is involved in connecting the olfactory system with the opposite side, by means of the *anterior commissure.* Another nuclear area is the *olfactory tubercle,* located at the posterior end of the olfactory tract. Some fibers of the olfactory tract form an intermediate stria that connects with this olfactory tubercle.

It is best to remember only the lateral tract as the principal tract of the olfactory system. It apparently has cortical tissue along its course for the termination of some olfactory fibers. The lateral tract ends in the cortex of the *uncal area* (see Figs. 4 and 5), with some of the fibers terminating in an adjacent part of the *amygdaloid nucleus* (see Figs. 71 and 72). The olfactory system terminates directly in primary olfactory areas of the cortex without a thalamic relay.

OLFACTORY CONNECTIONS

The connections of the olfactory system involve limbic cortex. These are called *secondary olfactory areas* and include the cortex in the anterior portion of the parahippocampal gyrus, an area that has been referred to as *entorhinal cortex.* (The term *rhinencephalon* refers to the olfactory parts of the CNS, the "smell brain".) This input of olfactory information into the limbic system makes sense if one remembers that one of the functions of the limbic system is procreation of the species. Smell is important in many species for mating behavior and for identification of the nest and territory.

Olfactory influences may spread to other parts of the limbic system, including the amygdala and the septal region. The connection with the septal region is carried in a band of fibers identifiable in detailed studies of the brain—the *diagonal band* (of Broca; see Figs. 82A and 82B). (This structure need not be remembered in an introductory course.) Through these various connections, information may reach the dorsomedial nucleus of the thalamus.

Smell is an interesting sensory system. We have all had the experience of a particular smell evoking a flood of memories, often associated with strong emotional overtones. This simply demonstrates the extensive connections that the olfactory system has with components of the limbic system and therefore with other parts of the brain.

One form of epilepsy often has a significant olfactory aura (which precedes the seizure itself). In such cases, the "trigger" area is often the orbitofrontal cortex. A significant association bundle interconnects this part of the frontal lobe with the anterior parts of the temporal lobe—the *uncinate bundle.* This particular form of epilepsy has unfortunately been given the name *uncinate fits.*

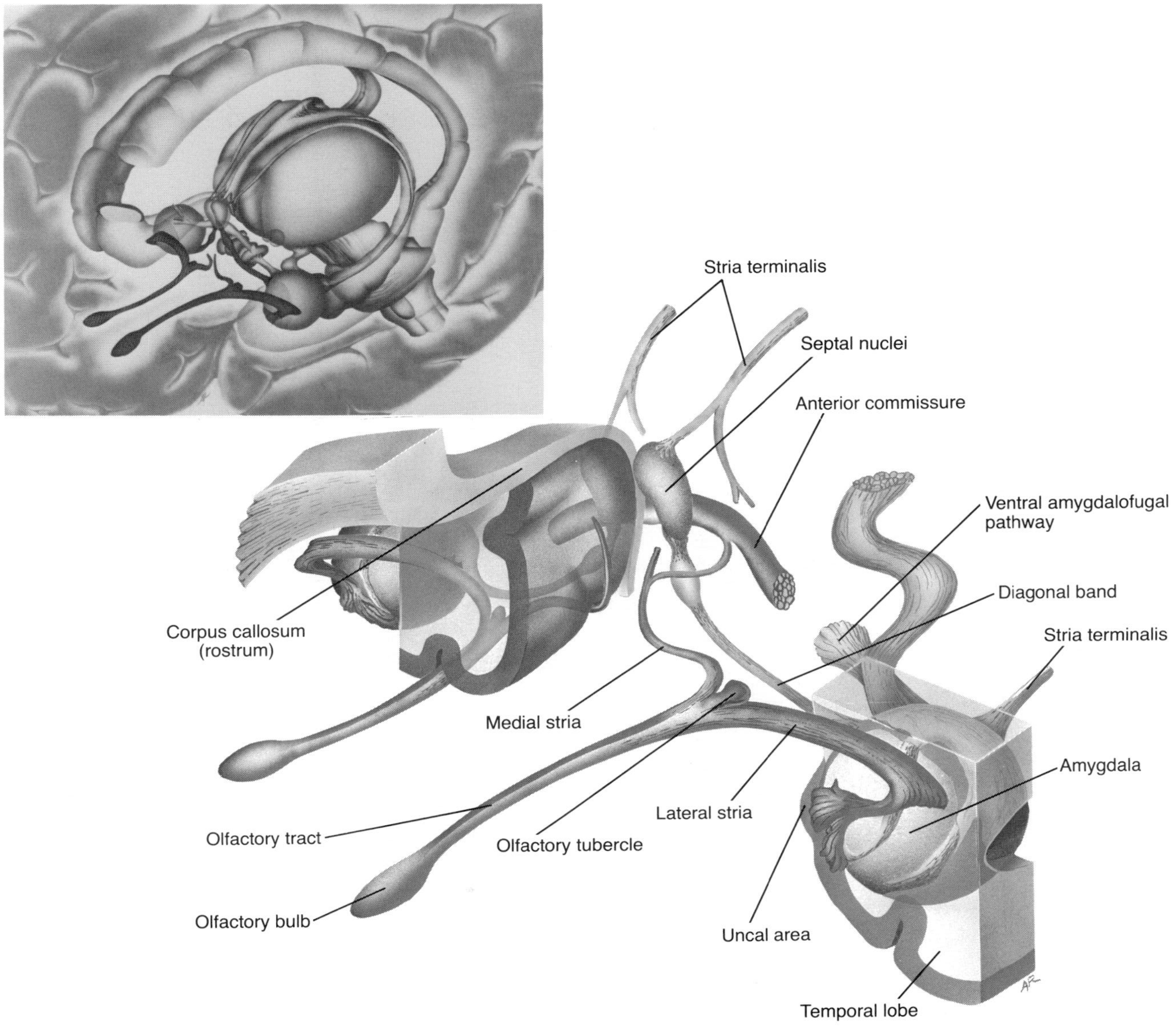

Stria terminalis

Septal nuclei

Anterior commissure

Ventral amygdalofugal pathway

Diagonal band

Stria terminalis

Amygdala

Temporal lobe

Uncal area

Lateral stria

Olfactory tubercle

Medial stria

Corpus callosum (rostrum)

Olfactory tract

Olfactory bulb

FIGURE 81

FIGURE 82A   # Basal Forebrain I

LIMBIC DIAGRAM (INSET)

The basal forebrain is an area that lies above the anterior perforated space and below the anterior commissure, lateral to the hypothalamus. The *anterior perforated space* can be located on the inferior surface of the brain where the olfactory tract ends and divides into medial and lateral striae (see Figs. 4 and 81). This is also the location where a number of blood vessels, the striate arteries, penetrate the brain substance—hence the name perforated.

BASAL FOREBRAIN STRUCTURES

The basal forebrain is the area previously called the *substantia innominata*. Inclusion of this region as part of the limbic system is still somewhat tentative. The ventral amygdalofugal pathway courses through this area (see Figs. 71, 72, and 81). It also contains a group of diverse structures, some of which are shown in this diagram and some in the next illustration. These include:

- the ventral portions of the putamen and globus pallidus—namely, the *ventral striatum* and *ventral pallidum*
- groups of cells that are continuous with the amygdala, now called the *extended amygdala*
- clusters of large cells that are cholinergic and that have been collectively called the *basal nucleus* (of Meynert)
- the *nucleus accumbens*, which may include a number of diverse neurons within its boundaries

The penetrating striate arteries are also shown in this region, supplying parts of the basal ganglia and internal capsule (discussed with Fig. 17).

VENTRAL AMYGDALOFUGAL PATHWAY

The ventral pathway from the amygdala (see Fig. 72) travels through this region, with part of it going to the hypothalamus and part to the dorsomedial nucleus of the thalamus (not shown here; see Fig. 80).

VENTRAL STRIATUM AND VENTRAL PALLIDUM

The ventral part of the striatum (the putamen) receives input from limbic cortical areas, as well as a dopaminergic pathway from a group of dopamine-containing cells in the midbrain. The information is then relayed to the ventral pallidum (both parts of the globus pallidus are seen on the left side of the diagram). This area has a significant projection to the dorsomedial nucleus of the thalamus (and hence to prefrontal cortex). The overall organization is therefore similar to that of the dorsal parts of the basal ganglia, although the sites of relay and termination are different.

NUCLEUS ACCUMBENS

This nucleus contains neurons that are part of the basal ganglia and other, possibly limbic neurons (see Fig. 15). It has many of the connections of the ventral striatum as well as those of the extended amygdala. Its functional contribution is still unknown, although it might be the neural area that becomes activated in situations that involve reward and punishment, integrating certain cognitive aspects of the situation with the emotional component.

OTHER STRUCTURES

Included with this diagram is a somewhat obscure limbic pathway, the diagonal band (of Broca), which connects the amygdaloid nucleus with the septal nuclei. As noted (see Fig. 81), it is probably part of the olfactory pathways. The extended amygdala and the cholinergic neurons are seen and discussed with the next illustration.

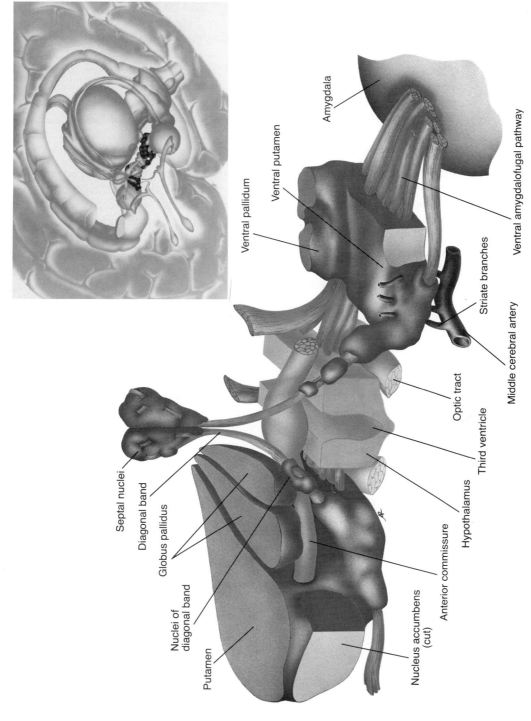

Septal nuclei

Diagonal band

Globus pallidus

Nuclei of diagonal band

Putamen

Ventral pallidum

Ventral putamen

Amygdala

Ventral amygdalofugal pathway

Striate branches

Middle cerebral artery

Optic tract

Third ventricle

Hypothalamus

Anterior commissure

Nucleus accumbens (cut)

FIGURE 82A

203

FIGURE 82B   # Basal Forebrain II

This is a more detailed illustration of the region of the basal forebrain.

EXTENDED AMYGDALA

A group of cells extends medially from the amygdaloid nucleus and follows the ventral pathway (the ventral amygdalofugal pathway; see Figs. 71 to 73) through this basal fore-brain region. It receives a variety of inputs from the limbic cortical areas and from other parts of the amygdala. Its output projects to the hypothalamus and to autonomic areas of the brain stem, thereby influencing neuroendocrine, somatomotor, and autonomic activities.

The various connections of these neurons may help to account for some of the symptoms seen clinically with seizures initiated in this area of the brain (discussed with Fig. 72).

CHOLINERGIC NEURONS

These are rather large neurons found in clusters throughout this region. (They are the darker cell groups in the illustration.) Although they receive input from the extended amygdala, the exact sources of additional input are not yet known. These cells project to widespread areas of the prefrontal cortex, providing that area with cholinergic innervation.

Several years ago, a depletion of acetylcholine was reported in the frontal lobe areas in patients with *Alzheimer's disease*. Subsequent reports indicated that this was accompanied by a loss of these cholinergic cells in the basal forebrain. Many thought that the "cause" of Alzheimer's disease had been uncovered—a cellular degeneration of a unique group of cells and a neurotransmitter deficit. (The model for this way of thinking is Parkinson's disease.) These reports were followed immediately be several therapeutic trials using medication to boost the acetylcholine levels of the brain.

It is currently thought that cortical degeneration is the primary event in Alzheimer's disease, often starting in the parietal areas of the brain. According to this postulate, the eventual loss of the target neurons in the prefrontal cortex, the site of termination for the cholinergic neurons, would be followed, presumably, by the degeneration of the cholinergic cells of the basal forebrain. Despite this altered way of looking at the data, therapeutic intervention to boost the cholinergic levels of the brain is still being used by some, particularly in the early stages of this tragic human disease.

In summary, the region of the basal forebrain has important links between parts of the limbic system and other parts of the brain. There is also a major output to the prefrontal cortex from the cholinergic neurons in this region. As noted, the prefrontal cortex is considered to be the forebrain component of the limbic system. The basal forebrain is thus thought to have a profound influence on basic drives and emotions, as well as higher cognitive functions that have an emotional component.

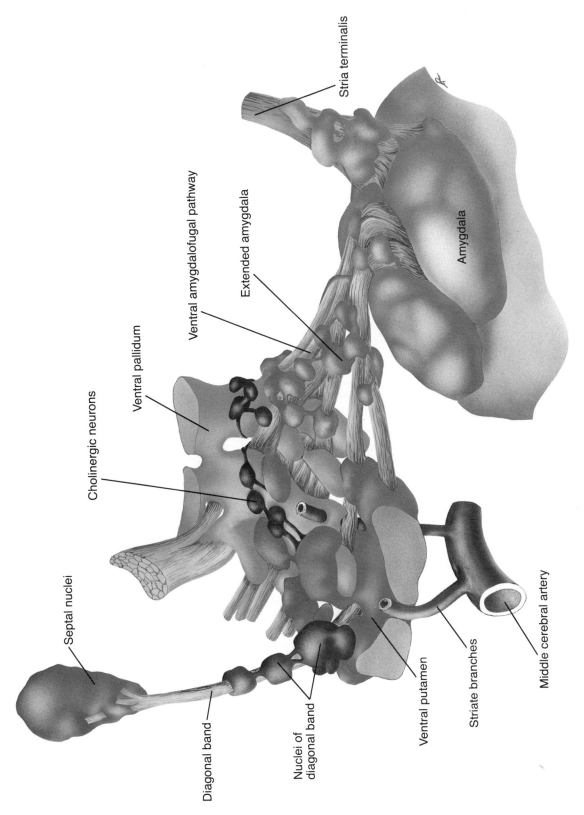

Stria terminalis

Amygdala

Ventral amygdalofugal pathway

Extended amygdala

Ventral pallidum

Cholinergic neurons

Septal nuclei

Diagonal band

Nuclei of
diagonal band

Ventral putamen

Striate branches

Middle cerebral artery

FIGURE 82B

205

Synthesis

At the beginning of this section, the idea of a limbic system was introduced and related to the notion of an emotional brain (see Introduction). The study of the structures and circuits, in some detail, has shown how one part of the limbic system influences another part, often involving a circuit or "loop." It is now appropriate to review how the limbic system fits the definition of "emotional brain" and how it influences or causes alterations in our behavior, in our physiologic state, and in our mental state (our mood, or the way we "feel" or react).

Although it is somewhat difficult to identify what each particular cortical area or nucleus of the limbic system does, it is easier to step back and consider globally how the limbic system fulfills its functions. This can be assessed by examining which parts of the brain receive input directly from limbic structures. The limbic pathways seem to terminate mainly in the following areas: the cortex, the midbrain, and the pituitary.

CORTEX (PREFRONTAL, CINGULATE AND PARAHIPPOCAMPAL)

The prefrontal cortex is currently described as the chief executive part of the brain. This large cortical association area is implicated in all kinds of behavior, from planning activities to reactions to situations. It is reciprocally connected to widespread areas of the brain. It is therefore quite consistent to view this part of the brain as the key area involved in the behavioral aspect of emotional reactions, working in concert with the basal ganglia (the ventral portions). Other parts, mainly the orbitofrontal regions, seem to be implicated in the alterations in our "mood," or mental state (our emotional tone).

The cingulate cortex, particularly its anterior portion, has recently been shown by positron emission tomography (PET) studies to be involved in attention. This would be consistent with the view that one of the functions of the limbic system is to alert the organism to matters of significance, either for survival or for satisfying the various "needs." In addition, the cingulate gyrus has connections with the prefrontal cortex and other cortical areas.

The parahippocampal gyrus communicates extensively with wide areas of the cerebral cortex, particularly sensory cortical regions, as well as the cingulate gyrus. Through its heavy (reciprocal) connections with the hippocampal formation, it seems to play a particular role in memory function.

MIDBRAIN (LIMBIC MIDBRAIN)

Many of the limbic pathways terminate directly or via the hypothalamus in the midbrain reticular formation, renamed the *limbic midbrain* in this section. These two regions, the hypothalamus and the limbic midbrain, seem to be involved in organizing the homeostatic responses of the organism, including activities involved in temperature regulation and satisfying other drives (appetite, thirst, sexual). Many of these responses involve complex motor behavior (e.g., consider the actions of a person who is cold, hungry, or thirsty). In addition, it is via these pathways that the limbic system influences the autonomic changes that accompany many emotional states (changes in blood pressure, pulse, and respiration; sweating; activities of our gastrointestinal tract).

PITUITARY

Hormonal changes, both acute and chronic, accompany many emotional states, in addition to those related to such activities as reproduction and water regulation. One of the classic examples is the work of Dr. Hans Selye, showing the influence of chronic stress on the organism. Again, it is via the hypothalamus that regulatory hormones alter the activity of the anterior pituitary gland.

The limbic system therefore has a much greater influence than the simple mnemonic used in the introduction to this section.

This summary of limbic functions is in good agreement with the definition proposed at the outset—the limbic system is an interrelated group of cortical and subcortical structures involved in the regulation of the emotional state, with the accompanying behavioral, physiologic, and psychologic responses. Some of these emotional states would involve our consciousness, whereas others would be reflected in the way we "feel" or react, our "mood" as many would simply call this modulation of our emotional tone.

At the outset we proposed an idea as to why memory is associated with the limbic structures. The particular type of memory involves noting events and holding them in temporary storage, sometimes termed *episodic memory*. The simplest idea is that this type of memory originally developed to allow the organism time to react to various situations, utilizing previous experience and correlating this with the ongoing activities of the nervous system. Depending on the outcome, the memory is then transferred to permanent "storage." We, as humans, have evolved in such a way that we rely almost totally on this memory system in a world that is built around millions of bits of information. Perhaps modern technology will relieve us of some of this burden and allow our nervous system to be involved in more creative human and humane pursuits.

Glossary

Abducens nerve   Sixth cranial nerve (VI).

Accessory nerve   Eleventh cranial nerve (XI).

Afferent   Toward (sensory if toward the central nervous system).

Agnosia   Lack of ability to recognize the significance of sensory stimuli (auditory, visual, tactile).

Agraphia   Inability to express thoughts in writing owing to a central lesion.

Alexia   Loss of the power to grasp the meaning of written or printed words and sentences.

Allocortex   The phylogenetically older cerebral cortex, usually consisting of three layers; includes paleocortex and archicortex (e.g., cortex of hippocampal formation).

Ammon's horn   The hippocampus proper, which has an outline in transverse section suggestive of a ram's horn; also known as the cornu Ammonis.

Amygdala   The amygdaloid body, located in the temporal lobe of the cerebral hemisphere. It is a nucleus of the limbic system.

Angiogram   Display of blood vessels in vivo for diagnostic purposes, by using contrast medium injected into the vascular system, followed by x-rays.

Anopsia   A defect of vision.

Anterolateral system   Ascending spinothalamic tracts for pain and temperature (lateral) and nondiscriminative touch (anterior).

Antidromic   Relating to the propagation of an impulse along an axon in a direction that is the reverse of the normal or usual direction.

Aphasia   A defect of the power of expression by speech or of comprehending spoken or written language.

Apraxia   Inability to carry out purposeful movements in the absence of paralysis.

Arachnoid   The middle layer of the meninges, forming the outer boundary of the subarachnoid space.

Archicerebellum   A phylogenetically old part of the cerebellum, functioning in the maintenance of equilibrium; includes the flocculonodular lobe.

Archicortex   Three-layered cortex found within the limbic system; located mainly in the hippocampus proper and dentate gyrus of the hippocampal formation.

Area postrema   An area in the caudal part of the floor of the fourth ventricle, involved in vomiting.

Ascending tract   Central sensory pathway, usually from spinal cord to brain stem or thalamus.

Association fibers   Fibers connecting parts of the cerebral hemisphere on the same side.

Astereognosis   Loss of ability to recognize objects or to appreciate their form by touching or feeling them.

Astrocyte   A type of neuroglial cell.

Asynergy   Disturbance of the proper sequencing in the contraction of muscles, at the proper moment and of the proper degree, so that the act cannot be executed accurately.

Ataxia   A loss of muscle coordination, with irregularity of muscle action.

Athetosis   An affliction of the nervous system, caused by degenerative changes in the basal ganglia, characterized by bizarre, writhing movements, especially of the fingers and toes.

Autonomic   Autonomic nervous system; usually taken to mean the efferent or motor innervation of viscera.

Autonomic nervous system   Visceral innervation; sympathetic and parasympathetic divisions.

Axon   Efferent process of a neuron conducting impulses to other neurons or to muscle fibers (striated and smooth) and gland cells.

Basal ganglia (nuclei)   Nuclei involved in motor control; includes the caudate, putamen and globus pallidus (the lentiform nucleus), the subthalamus, and the substantia nigra.

Basilar artery   The major artery supplying the brain stem and cerebellum, formed by the two vertebral arteries.

Brachium   As used in the central nervous system, denotes a large bundle of fibers connecting one part with another (e.g., brachium associated with the inferior colliculus).

Bradykinesia   Abnormal slowness of movements.

Brain stem   In the mature human brain, usually denotes the medulla, pons, and midbrain.

Bulb   Referred at one time to the medulla oblongata but, in the context of "corticobulbar tract," refers to the brain stem in which motor nuclei of cranial nerves are located.

CAT, or CT scan   Abbreviation for computed axial tomography (CAT) or computed tomography (CT): a diagnostic imaging technique.

Cauda equina   "Horse's tail": the lower lumbar, sacral, and coccygeal spinal nerves as they lie in the vertebral canal, below the level of the spinal cord.

Caudal   Toward the tail, or hindmost part of the neuraxis.

Caudate nucleus   Part of the neostriatum, so named because it has a long extension or tail.

Central nervous system (CNS)   Brain and spinal cord.

Cerebellar peduncle   Inferior, middle, and superior; fiber tracts linking cerebellum and brain stem.

Cerebellum   The little brain. A large part of the brain with motor functions, situated in the posterior cranial fossa.

Cerebral aqueduct (of Sylvius)   Passage through the midbrain, part of the ventricular system.

Cerebral peduncle   Descending cortical fibers in the "basal" portion of the midbrain; often includes the substantia nigra.

Cerebrospinal fluid (CSF)   The fluid in the ventricles and in the subarachnoid space.

Cerebrum   The principal portion of the brain, including the diencephalon and cerebral hemispheres, but not the brain stem and cerebellum.

Cervical   Referring to the neck region.

Chorda tympani   Part of the seventh cranial nerve (VII) (see Facial nerve).

Chordotomy   Cutting of the spinothalamic tract for intractable pain (tractotomy). Also spelled cordotomy.

Chorea   A disorder characterized by irregular, spasmodic, involuntary movements of the limbs or facial muscles; attributed to degenerative changes in the neostriatum.

Choroid   A delicate membrane. Choroid plexuses are found in the ventricles of the brain.

Choroid plexus   Vascular structures "secreting" cerebrospinal fluid into the ventricles.

Cingulum   A bundle of association fibers in the white matter of the cingulate gyrus on the medial surface of the cerebral hemisphere.

Circle of Willis Anastomosis between internal cartoid and basilar arteries in the region of the optic chiasm, above the pituitary gland.

Cistern(a) Expanded portion of the subarachnoid space, containing cerebrospinal fluid.

Claustrum A thin sheet of gray matter, of unknown function, situated between the lentiform nucleus and the insula.

CNS Abbreviation for central nervous system.

Colliculus A small elevation or mound; superior and inferior colliculi comprising the tectum of the midbrain; facial colliculus in the floor of the fourth ventricle.

Commissure A joining together; a bundle of nerve fibers passing from one side to the other in the brain or spinal cord.

Contralateral On the opposite side.

Corona radiata Fibers radiating from the internal capsule to various parts of the cerebral cortex.

Corpus callosum The main neocortical commissure of the cerebral hemispheres.

Corpus striatum Caudate, putamen, and globus pallidus, nuclei inside the cerebral hemisphere, with motor function; the basal ganglia.

Cortex Outer layer of gray matter (neurons and neuropil) of the cerebral hemispheres and cerebellum.

Corticobulbar tract Descending tract connecting the motor cortex with the motor cranial nerve nuclei of the brain stem.

Corticospinal tract Descending tract, from the motor cortex to the anterior (ventral) horn cells of the spinal cord.

Cranial nerve nuclei Collections of cells in the brain stem giving rise to or receiving fibers from cranial nerves; may be sensory or motor.

Cranial nerves Twelve pairs of nerves, ten of which arise from the brain stem, innervating structures of the head and neck.

Crus cerebri Basal part of the cerebral peduncle of the midbrain, containing corticospinal and corticobulbar tracts, and corticopontine fibers; separated from the dorsal part by the substantia nigra. (Also called the basis pedunculi.)

CSF Abbreviation for cerebrospinal fluid.

Cuneatus Sensory tract (fasciculus cuneatus) of the dorsal column of the spinal cord; nucleus cuneatus of the medulla.

Decussation The point of crossing of paired tracts. Examples are decussations of the pyramids, medial lemnisci, and superior cerebellar peduncles.

Dendrite Receptive process of a neuron.

Dentate (toothed) Dentate nucleus of the cerebellum; dentate gyrus of the hippocampal formation.

Descending tract Central motor pathway (e.g., from the brain to the spinal cord).

Diencephalon Part of the cerebrum, consisting of the thalamus, epithalamus, subthalamus, and hypothalamus.

Diplopia Double vision.

Dorsal column Fasciculus (tract) gracilis and fasciculus cuneatus of the spinal cord; pathways for discriminative touch and conscious proprioception.

Dorsal root Afferent sensory component of a mixed spinal nerve.

Dura Dura mater, the thick external layer of the meninges.

Dural venous sinuses Large venous channels for draining blood from the brain; run in the dura mater.

Dyskinesia Abnormality of motor function, characterized by involuntary, purposeless movements.

Dysmetria Disturbance of the ability to control the range of movement in muscular action.

Efferent   Away from (motor if away from the central nervous system).

Emboliform   Emboliform nucleus of the cerebellum, one of the intracerebellar nuclei.

Entorhinal   The entorhinal area is the anterior part of the parahippocampal gyrus of the temporal lobe adjacent to the uncus. It is involved with olfaction (smell).

Ependyma   Lining epithelium of the ventricles of the brain and of the central canal of the spinal cord.

Epithalamus   A region of the diencephalon above the thalamus; includes the habenula and pineal body.

External capsule   White matter superficial to the lentiform nucleus.

Extrapyramidal system   In broadest terms, consists of all motor parts of the central nervous system except the pyramidal (corticospinal) system. "Extrapyramidal system" is subject to various interpretations and is more often used clinically than anatomically.

Facial nerve   Seventh cranial nerve (VII) (see Chorda tympani).

Falx   Two of the dural partitions in the cranial cavity, the large falx cerebri between the cerebral hemispheres, and the small falx cerebelli.

Fasciculus   A tract or bundle of nerve fibers.

Fasciculus cuneatus   Ascending tract for conscious proprioception and discriminative touch, part of the dorsal column of the spinal cord.

Fasciculus gracilis   Ascending tract for conscious proprioception and discriminative touch, part of the dorsal column of the spinal cord.

Fastigial   Fastigial nucleus of the cerebellum, one of the intracerebellar nuclei.

Fiber   See Axon.

Fimbria   A band of nerve fibers along the medial edge of the hippocampus, continuing as the fornix.

Flocculus   Part of the archicerebellum.

Folium   (plural = folia) A flat leaflike fold of the cerebellar cortex.

Foramen   An opening, aperture.

Foramen of Luschka   Lateral foramen (of fourth ventricle).

Foramen of Magendie   Median foramen (of fourth ventricle).

Forebrain   Anterior division (vesicle) of embryonic brain; cerebrum and diencephalon of the adult brain.

Fornix   The efferent subcortical tract of the hippocampal formation, arching over the thalamus and terminating in the mammillary nucleus of the hypothalamus and in the septal region.

Fourth ventricle   Cavity in the hindbrain, containing cerebrospinal fluid.

Frontal lobe   Part of the cerebral hemisphere.

Funiculus   A large aggregation of white matter in the spinal cord; may contain several tracts.

Ganglion   (plural = ganglia) A swelling composed of nerve cells, as in dorsal root ganglion and sympathetic ganglion. Also used inappropriately for certain regions of gray matter in the brain (e.g., basal ganglia of the cerebral hemisphere).

Geniculate bodies   Nuclei of the thalamus—lateral and medial; relay centers for visual (lateral) and auditory (medial) pathways.

Genu   (knee) Anterior bend of the corpus callosum; genu of the facial nerve; genu of the internal capsule.

Glial cells   Supporting cells in the central nervous system (astrocytes and oligodendrocytes).

Globus pallidus   Medial part of the lentiform nucleus of the corpus striatum; efferent part of the basal ganglia (paleostriatum).

Glossopharyngeal nerve   Ninth cranial nerve (IX).

Gracilis   Sensory tract (fasciculus gracilis) of the dorsal column of the spinal cord; nucleus gracilis of the medulla.

Granule   Used to denote small neurons, such as granule cells of the cerebellar cortex and stellate cells of the cerebral cortex; hence granular cell layers of both cortices.

Gray matter   Nervous tissue, mainly nerve cell bodies and adjacent neuropil; looks "grayish" after fixation in formalin.

Gyrus   (plural = gyri) A convoluted fold of a cerebral hemisphere.

Habenula   A small nuclear area in the epithalamus, adjacent to the posterior end of the roof of the third ventricle.

Hemiballismus   An uncontrolled flinging movement of one or both limbs on one side of the body, caused by a destructive lesion involving the contralateral subthalamic nucleus.

Hemiplegia   Paralysis of one side of the body.

Hindbrain   Posterior division of the embryonic brain; pons and medulla oblongata and cerebellum of the adult brain.

Hippocampus, or hippocampus "proper"   Specialized area of phylogenetically old (3-layered) cortex in the floor of the inferior horn of the lateral ventricle, in the temporal lobe; part of the limbic system, but involved mostly with the formation of new memories.

Hydrocephalus   Excessive accumulation of cerebrospinal fluid in the brain.

Hypoglossal nerve   Twelfth cranial nerve (XII).

Hypothalamus   A region of the diencephalon that serves as the main controlling center of homeostasis and of the autonomic nervous system; is involved in several limbic circuits. Also regulates the activity of the pituitary gland.

Infundibulum   (funnel) Infundibular stem of the neurohypophysis, the neural part of the pituitary gland.

Innervation   Nerve supply, sensory or motor.

Insula   (island) Cerebral cortex concealed from surface view and lying at the bottom of the lateral sulcus. Also called the island of Reil.

Internal capsule   White matter between the lentiform nucleus and the thalamus and the head of the caudate nucleus, consisting of anterior limb, genu, and posterior limb.

Internal carotid artery   One of the arteries supplying the brain.

Interventricular foramen   (of Monro) Opening from the lateral into the third ventricle.

Ipsilateral   On the same side.

Isocortex   Cerebral cortex having six layers (neocortex).

Kinesthesia   The sense of perception of movement.

Lacunae   Irregularly shaped venous "lakes" or channels draining into the superior sagittal sinus.

Lateral foramen   Foramen of Luschka, opening in the lateral recess of the fourth ventricle for escape of cerebrospinal fluid into the subarachnoid space surrounding the brain stem. There are two openings (foramina), one on each side.

Lateral ventricle   Cavity, one in each cerebral hemisphere, containing cerebrospinal fluid. Also known as ventricles I and II.

Lemniscus   Used to designate a bundle of nerve fibers in the central nervous system (e.g., medial lemniscus and lateral lemniscus).

Lentiform   (lens-shaped) Lentiform nucleus, a component of the basal ganglia. Also called lenticular nucleus. Composed of the putamen and the globus pallidus.

Leptomeninges   Arachnoid and pia mater.

Limbic system   Parts of the brain associated with emotional behavior.

Limbus (a border) Limbic lobe: a C-shaped configuration of cortex on the medial surface of the cerebral hemisphere, consisting of the subcallosal gyri of the septal region and the cingulate and parahippocampal gyri.

Locus ceruleus A small nucleus of the pons on each side of the floor of the fourth ventricle; contains pigment.

Lower motor neurons Anterior horn cells (and their axons) of the spinal cord, or equivalent cells in the motor cranial nerve nuclei.

Lumbar Referring to the lower back region.

Mammillary Mammillary bodies: nuclei that are seen as small swellings on the ventral surface of the hypothalamus. Also spelled mamillary.

Massa intermedia A bridge of gray matter connecting the thalami of the two sides across the third ventricle; present in 70% of human brains. Also called the interthalamic adhesion.

Medial lemniscus Brain stem portion of sensory pathway for discriminative touch and conscious proprioception, after synapse in nucleus gracilis and nucleus cuneatus.

Medial longitudinal fasciculus (MLF) A tract throughout the brain stem and cervical spinal cord that interconnects visual and vestibular input with movements of the eyes and the head and neck.

Median foramen Foramen of Magendie, opening in the roof of the fourth ventricle into the cisterna magna of the subarachnoid space, below the cerebellum and behind the medulla.

Medulla Medulla oblongata: the caudal portion of the brain stem.

Meninges Covering layers of the central nervous system, composed of connective tissue (dura, arachnoid, and pia).

Mesencephalon The midbrain: the upper portion of the brain stem.

Metathalamus The medial and lateral geniculate bodies (nuclei).

Midbrain The middle division of the embryonic brain, part of the adult brain stem (also known as the mesencephalon).

Mnemonic Pertaining to memory.

Modality A type of sensation (e.g., discriminative touch, vision).

Motor To do with movement or response.

MRI Abbreviation for magnetic resonance imaging, a diagnostic imaging technique (see NMR).

Myelin The layers of lipid and protein substances composing a sheath around nerve fibers that is important for rapid nerve conduction.

Myelin sheath Covering of a nerve fiber; part of the Schwann cell (peripheral nervous system) or oligodendrocyte (central nervous system).

Neocerebellum The phylogenetically newest part of the cerebellum, present in mammals and especially well developed in humans; consists of the lateral lobes. Ensures smooth muscle action in the finer voluntary movements and involved in motor planning.

Neocortex Six-layered cortex, characteristic of mammals and constituting most of the cerebral cortex in humans.

Neostriatum The phylogenetically newer part of the basal ganglia consisting of the caudate nucleus and putamen; the striatum.

Nerve fiber Neuronal cell process, plus sheathing cells, plus myelin if present.

Neuraxis The straight longitudinal axis of the embryonic or primitive neural tube, bent in later evolution and development.

Neuroglia Accessory or interstitial cells of the central nervous system; includes astrocytes, oligodendrocytes, microglial cells, and ependymal cells.

Neuron   The morphological unit of the nervous system, consisting of the nerve cell body and its processes (dendrites and axon).

Neuropil   A complex net of nerve cell processes and synapses occupying the areas between cell bodies in the gray matter.

NMR   Abbreviation for nuclear magnetic resonance, also known as magnetic resonance imaging (MRI); a diagnostic imaging method.

Nociceptive   Responsive to injurious stimuli.

Node of Ranvier   Gap in the myelin sheath between two successive Schwann cells or oligodendrocytes.

Nucleus   (plural = nuclei) An aggregation of nerve cells within the CNS.

Nystagmus   An involuntary oscillation of the eyes.

Occipital lobe   Part of the cerebral hemisphere.

Oculomotor nerve   Third cranial nerve (III).

Olfactory nerve   First cranial nerve (I).

Oligodendrocyte   A neuroglial cell; forms the myelin sheath in the central nervous system in the same manner as the Schwann cell in peripheral nerves.

Optic chiasm(a)   Partial crossing of the optic nerves, after which the optic tracts are formed.

Optic nerve   Second cranial nerve (II).

Paleocerebellum   A phylogenetically old part of the cerebellum functioning in postural changes and locomotion; consists of anterior lobe, intermediate zone, and most of the vermis.

Paleocortex   Phylogenetically older cerebral cortex consisting of three to five layers.

Paleostriatum   Globus pallidus; the phylogenetically older and efferent part of the basal ganglia (also called the pallidum).

Paralysis   Loss of voluntary action.

Paraplegia   Paralysis of both legs and the lower part of the trunk.

Paresis   Partial paralysis (denotes a weakness).

Parietal lobe   Part of the cerebral hemisphere.

Pathway   A chain of functionally interconnected neurons making a connection between one region of the central nervous system and another; a tract or tracts and the associated nuclei, e.g., visual pathway.

Peduncle   A thick stalk or stem; bundle of nerve fibers.

Perikaryon   The cytoplasm surrounding the nucleus of a neuron. Sometimes refers to the cell body of a neuron.

Peripheral nervous system (PNS)   Nerve roots, nerves, and ganglia (sensory and autonomic) outside the central nervous system.

PET   Abbreviation for positron emission tomography; a technique used to visualize areas of the living brain that become "activated" under certain task conditions.

Pia mater   The thin, innermost layer of the meninges, attached to the surface of the brain and spinal cord; forms the inner boundary of the subarachnoid space.

Pineal   Pertaining to the pineal body; also called the pineal gland (part of epithalamus).

Plexus   An arrangement of interwoven vessels or nerves that forms a network.

PNS   Abbreviation for peripheral nervous system.

Pons   (bridge) That part of the brain stem that lies between the medulla and the midbrain; appears to constitute a bridge between the right and left halves of the cerebellum.

Proprioception   The sense of body position (conscious or unconscious).

Proprioceptor   One of the sensory endings in muscles, tendons, and joints; provides information concerning movement and position of body parts (proprioception).

Ptosis   Drooping of the upper eyelid.

Pulvinar   The posterior nuclear area of the thalamus; functionally involved with vision.

Putamen   The larger and lateral part of the lentiform nucleus; part of the neostriatum of the basal ganglia, with the caudate nucleus.

Pyramidal system   Corticospinal (and corticobulbar) tracts. So called because the corticospinal tracts occupy the pyramid-shaped areas on the ventral surface of the medulla. The term pyramidal tract refers specifically to the corticospinal tract.

Quadriplegia   Paralysis affecting the four limbs. Also called tetraplegia.

Raphe   An anatomical structure in the midline. In the brain, several raphe nuclei of the reticular formation are in the midline of the medulla, pons, and midbrain.

Red nucleus   Nucleus in the midbrain (sometimes has a reddish color in fresh material).

Reticular   Pertaining to or resembling a net.

Reticular formation   Diffuse nervous tissue network in the brain stem; a group of nuclei throughout the brain stem.

Rhinencephalon   Refers in humans to components of the olfactory system (smell).

Rostral   Toward the nose, or the most anterior end of the neuraxis.

Rostrum   Recurved anterior portion of the corpus callosum.

Rubrospinal tract   Descending tract from the red nucleus of the midbrain to the spinal cord.

Saccadic   (to jerk) Extremely quick movements of the eyes in altering the direction of gaze.

Sacral   Referring to the pelvic region.

Schwann cell   Sheathing cell of peripheral nerve fibers, responsible for formation and maintenance of myelin.

Secretomotor   Motor nerve supply to a gland.

Sensory   To do with receiving information from the external or internal environment.

Septal region   An area ventral to the genu and rostrum of the corpus callosum on the medial aspect of the frontal lobe; includes the subcallosal gyri and the septal nuclei; part of the limbic system.

Septum pellucidum   A triangular double membrane separating the frontal horns of the lateral ventricles. Situated in the median plane, it fills the interval between the corpus callosum and the fornix.

Somatic   Used in neurology to denote the body, exclusive of the viscera (as in somatic efferent neurons supplying the skeletal musculature).

Somatic senses   The senses of touch, pain, temperature, pressure, proprioception, and vibration.

Somesthetic   The consciousness of having a body. Somesthetic senses are the general senses of pain, temperature, touch, pressure, position, movement, and vibration.

Special senses   The senses of sight, hearing, balance, taste (gustatory), and smell (olfactory).

Spinocerebellar tracts   Ascending tracts, anterior and posterior, for unconscious proprioception to the cerebellum.

Spinothalamic tracts   Ascending tracts for pain and temperature (lateral) and nondiscriminative touch and pressure (anterior); form the anterolateral system.

Splenium   The thickened posterior portion of the corpus callosum.

Strabismus   (a squint) A constant lack of parallelism of the visual axes of the eyes.

Stria terminalis   A slender strand of fibers running along with the tail and body of the caudate nucleus. Originating in the amygdaloid body, most of the fibers end in the septal region and hypothalamus.

Striatum   The phylogenetically more recent part of the basal ganglia (neostriatum), consisting of the caudate nucleus and the putamen (lateral portion of the lentiform nucleus).

Subarachnoid space   The space between the arachnoid and pia mater, containing cerebrospinal fluid.

Subcortical   Not in the cerebral cortex, i.e., at a functionally or evolutionarily "lower" level in the central nervous system; also refers to white matter of the cerebral hemispheres.

Subiculum   Transitional cortex between that of the parahippocampal gyrus and the hippocampus proper; part of the hippocampal formation.

Substantia gelatinosa   A column of small neurons at the apex of the dorsal gray horn throughout the spinal cord.

Substantia nigra   A large nucleus with motor functions in the midbrain, consisting of two parts (pars compacta and pars reticularis); many of the constituent cells in the pars compacta contain dark melanin pigment. These neurons degenerate in Parkinson's disease.

Subthalamus   Region of the diencephalon beneath the thalamus, containing fiber tracts and the subthalamic nucleus.

Sulcus   (plural = sulci) Groove between adjacent gyri.

Synapse   An area of structural and functional specialization between neurons where transmission of neural messages occurs. In the human brain, most synapses are chemical and involve excitation, inhibition, or modulation.

Syringomyelia   A condition characterized by central cavitation of the spinal cord and gliosis around the cavity.

Tectum   Roof of the midbrain, consisting of the paired superior and inferior colliculi.

Tegmentum   The "core area" of the brain stem, between the ventricle (or aqueduct) and the corticospinal tract; contains the reticular formation, cranial nerve and other nuclei, and various tracts.

Telencephalon   Rostral part of embryonic forebrain; primarily the cerebral hemisphere of the adult brain.

Temporal lobe   Part of the cerebral hemisphere.

Tentorium   The tentorium cerebelli is a dural partition between the occipital lobes of the cerebral hemispheres and the cerebellum.

Thalamus   A major portion of the diencephalon with sensory, motor, and integrative functions.

Third ventricle   Cavity in the diencephalon, containing cerebrospinal fluid.

Tomography   Sectional roentgenography. Computerized (or computed) tomography (CT) is a valuable diagnostic technique.

Tract   A bundle of nerve fibers within the central nervous system, with a common origin and termination, e.g., optic tract.

Trapezoid body   Transverse crossing fibers of the auditory pathway situated in the ventral portion of the tegmentum of the pons.

Trigeminal nerve   Fifth cranial nerve (V).

Trigeminothalamic tracts   Ascending tracts for sensations from the face (to the thalamus).

Trochlear nerve   Fourth cranial nerve (IV).

Uncus   The hooked-back portion of the rostral end of the parahippocampal gyrus of the temporal lobe, constituting a landmark for the lateral olfactory area; the amygdaloid nucleus lies deep to this area.

Upper motor neuron   Cell in the motor cortex or other motor areas in the brain or brain stem connected by descending tract to lower motor neurons.

Vagus nerve   Tenth cranial nerve (X).

Velum   (plural = vela) A membranous structure. The superior and inferior medullary vela form the roof of the fourth ventricle.

Ventral root   Efferent motor component of a mixed spinal nerve.

Ventricles   Cerebrospinal fluid (CSF) filled cavities inside the brain.

Vermis   Unpaired midline portion of the cerebellum between the cerebellar hemispheres.

Vertebral artery   An artery (one of a pair) supplying the spinal cord and the brain stem.

Vestibulocochlear nerve   Eighth cranial nerve (VIII) (acoustic nerve).

Vestibulospinal tract   Descending tract from the vestibular nuclei of the brain stem to the spinal cord; refers usually to the lateral vestibulospinal tract from the lateral vestibular nucleus.

Visceral   Referring to internal organs.

White matter   Nervous tissue made up mainly of nerve fibers (axons), some of which are myelinated; appears "whitish" after fixation in formalin.

Annotated Bibliography

This is a select reference list, with some commentary, to help guide the student to additional available texts, atlases, and videotapes. The emphasis is on recent publications.

Texts

Burt, A.M.: *Textbook of Neuroanatomy*. Philadelphia, W.B. Saunders, 1993.

A very good coverage of basic neuroanatomy. Includes some "physiological" sections and a chapter on the limbic system, as well as clinical correlations.

Carpenter, M.B.: *Core Text of Neuroanatomy*, 4th ed. Baltimore, Williams & Wilkins, 1991.

A detailed treatment of the subject matter by a highly respected author. Contains some excellent diagrams, many with color, and includes functional considerations.

Fitzgerald, M.J.T.: *Neuroanatomy: Basic and Clinical*, 2nd ed. London, Balliere Tindall, 1992.

A concise text, combining text and clinical aspects, with many illustrations.

Guyton, A.C.: *Basic Neuroscience: Anatomy and Physiology*, 2nd ed. Philadelphia, W.B. Saunders, 1991.

A concise explanation of the physiological aspects of the central nervous system. Contains many handy illustrations to amplify the text.

Kandel, E.R., Schwartz, J.H., Jessell, T.M.: *Principles of Neural Science*, 3rd ed. New York, Elsevier, 1991.

A thorough treatment of the functional (physiological) aspects of the nervous system. Suitable for graduate students and as a reference book for select topics.

Martin, J.H.: *Neuroanatomy: Text and Atlas*. New York, Elsevier, 1989.

A rather complete neuroanatomical text, with many illustrations, meant to serve as a companion text to Kandel, Schwartz, and Jessell. There is a small atlas section at the end of the text.

Noback, C.R., Strominger, N.L., Demarest, R.J.: *The Human Nervous System: Introduction and Review*, 4th ed. Philadelphia, Lea & Febiger, 1991.

A concise basic text of neuroanatomy, with many fine illustrations.

Nolte, J.: *The Human Brain*. 3rd ed. St. Louis, Mosby Year Book, 1993.

Another introductory text with a functional viewpoint and some interesting illustrations. A companion study guide is published separately.

Williams, P., Warwick, R.: *Functional Neuroanatomy of Man*. Philadelphia, W.B. Saunders, 1975.

The neurology section from the 35th edition of Gray's Anatomy. *Excellent anatomical reference (although dated) for the peripheral, autonomic, and central nervous systems.*

Wilson-Pauwels, L., Akesson, E.J., Stewart, P.A.: *Cranial Nerves: Anatomy and Clinical Comments*. Toronto, B.C. Decker, 1988.

A handy resource on the cranial nerves, with some very nice illustrations. Relatively complete and easy to follow.

Atlases

DeArmond, S.J., Fusco, M.M., Dewey, M.M.: *Structure of the Human Brain: A Photographic Atlas,* 2nd ed. New York, Oxford University Press, 1976.

A detailed atlas of the brain, both gross and microscopic, in all planes. No color material and no explanatory text. It is a good reference.

England, M.A., Wakely, J.: *Color Atlas of the Brain and Spinal Cord.* St. Louis, Mosby Year Book, 1991.

A very well illustrated atlas, with most of the photographs and sections in color. Very little in the way of text. Could be used to supplement a structured course.

Haines, D.E.: *Neuroanatomy: An Atlas of Structures, Sections and Systems,* 3rd ed. Baltimore, Urban & Schwarzenberg, 1991.

This is a relatively complete atlas of the nervous system, with many fine illustrations, particularly of the gross brain. Much detail is included in the brain stem cross sections. Explanatory text is available only with the functional diagrams.

Netter, F.H.: *The CIBA Collection of Medical Illustrations,* Volume I: Nervous System. Part I: Anatomy and Physiology, Summit, NJ, CIBA, 1983.

An excellent atlas containing drawings, in color, of the skull; the central, autonomic, and peripheral nervous systems; embryology; and some functional material. Well worth viewing.

Videotapes*

Hendelman, W.J.: *Interior of the Skull.* Chapel Hill, NC, Health Sciences Consortium, 1990.

Hendelman, W.J.: *The Gross Anatomy of the Human Brain Series.* Part I: The Hemispheres. Part II: Diencephalon, Brainstem and Cerebellum. Part III: Cerebrovascular System and Cerebrospinal Fluid. Part IV: The Limbic System. Chapel Hill, NC, Health Sciences Consortium, 1990.

These tapes are laboratory demonstrations of the anatomy, illustrated on actual specimens, with a narrative, each of approximately 25 minutes' duration. They have been prepared with the same teaching orientation as this ATLAS. The tapes can be used by students for self-study, particularly where specimens are not easily available; a study guide is included with each purchased tape. They have also been used to supplement a lecture, with an appropriate projection system onto a full-size screen. Recommended for purchase by a library or through an instructional media resource unit.

---

* Information regarding the purchase of these and other videotapes may be obtained from the Health Sciences Consortium, a nonprofit publishing cooperative dedicated to sharing instructional resources, 201 Silver Cedar Ct., Chapel Hill, NC 27514-1517; telephone (919) 942-8731, FAX (919) 942-3689.

Index

Note: Page numbers in *italics* refer to illustrations; page numbers followed by (d) refer to glossary definitions.